Vietnam War Nurses

ALSO BY PATRICIA RUSHTON

Gulf War Nurses:
Personal Accounts of 14 Americans,
1990–1991 and 2003–2010
(McFarland, 2011)

Vietnam War Nurses

Personal Accounts of 18 Americans

PATRICIA RUSHTON

McFarland & Company, Inc., Publishers
Jefferson, North Carolina, and London

LIBRARY OF CONGRESS CATALOGUING-IN-PUBLICATION DATA

Rushton, Patricia.
    Vietnam War nurses : personal accounts of 18 Americans /
Patricia Rushton.
        p.   cm.
    Includes bibliographical references and index.

    ISBN 978-0-7864-7352-6
    softcover : acid free paper ∞

    1. Vietnam War, 1961–1975—Medical care.   2. Vietnam
War, 1961–1975—Personal narratives, American.   3. United
States. Army Nurse Corps—Biography.   4. United States.
Army Nurse Corps—History—Vietnam War, 1961–1975.
5. United States—Armed Forces—Nurses—Biography.
6. Military nursing—United States—History—20th century.
7. Military nursing—Vietnam—History—20th century.
I. Title.
DS559.44.R87 2013
959.704'37—dc23   2013008754

BRITISH LIBRARY CATALOGUING DATA ARE AVAILABLE

On the cover: Lieutenant Commander Lou Ellen Bell (courtesy of
Lou Ellen Bell); incoming rockets (courtesy of Lou Ellen Bell);
background image (Stocktrek Images/Thinkstock)

Manufactured in the United States of America

McFarland & Company, Inc., Publishers
   Box 611, Jefferson, North Carolina 28640
   www.mcfarlandpub.com

Table of Contents

Introduction

The Vietnam War was my war. I joined because the Navy would pay for the last two years of my university nursing education and because the Navy recruiter, Sandy Kirkpatrick (whose account follows in this book), looked very sharp in her dress blues. Seeing the world didn't even cross my mind. I was just excited to see Pennsylvania and Philadelphia, the birthplace of American democracy, and the Liberty Bell, Independence Hall, Valley Forge and Gettysburg. There was something wonderful about telling folks I had joined the Navy. I didn't understand all the politics surrounding the reasons we were in Vietnam, but at a time when there was so much discussion about the right and wrong of the war, I was very proud to be serving my country providing nursing care to servicemen.

I finished my formal nursing education and went on active duty at Philadelphia Naval Hospital. It was there I learned about myself. I learned just how much I loved my family and believed in my faith. I learned to be a good nurse. I learned to organize the work and prioritize to get important things done in an appropriate order. I learned to be in charge, a trait that has shaped many of the decisions and actions in my life since then.

I am so grateful for my experience during the war in Vietnam. It is one of those experiences that made all the difference in my life. But this is not my story. That has been told in other places (Rushton, 2005). The stories that follow in this work tell about many aspects of nursing during the "Vietnam experience."

Brief History of the War in Vietnam

The war in Vietnam has been characterized as "America's War." Depending on the source, the United States was involved in the Vietnam experience from 1945 or 1950, when President Harry S. Truman provided aid and advisors to the French military, until 1975, during the administration of President Lyndon B. Johnson, when the American embassy was evacuated during the fall of Saigon. During that 25- to 30-year span, five U.S. presidents held office, 3,300,000 Americans served, 57,605 were killed and 303,700 were wounded.

The military involvement of the United States in Vietnam was initially to provide aid to the French, who were trying to maintain their Vietnamese colony and protect it from Vietnamese rebels led by Ho Chi Minh. President Dwight D. Eisenhower believed in the domino theory. According to Roarke, Eisenhower once said, "You have a row of dominoes set up. You knock over the first one, and what will happen to the last one is the certainty it will go over very quickly." Roarke also noted that Eisenhower warned, "The fall of Southeast Asia to communism could well be followed by the fall of Japan, Taiwan, and the Philippines." By 1954 the U.S. was providing 75 percent of the cost of the war to the French. Eisenhower did not provide troops to the French and France was defeated and signed a truce in 1954.

The truce created the countries of North and South Vietnam. John F. Kennedy ultimately supported South Vietnam in the conflict between the two nations, providing troops and materials. Johnson continued the support. Roarke commented that the numbers of troops and the resources committed to the war failed to defeat North Vietnam in its conquest to unite North and South Vietnam under a communist government, but they added the burden of intense conflict at home in the United States. Hundreds of thousands of Americans felt the war was immoral and futile and protested against it. Richard Nixon was president of the United States when the formal accord was signed in Paris in 1973 to end the war. However, the American embassy remained open and the U.S. continued to support South Vietnam with bombing in neighboring countries. In 1975 when the North Vietnamese entered and took over Saigon, the United States embassy staff and 150,000 South Vietnamese were evacuated in a massive and chaotic airlift.

The ability to fight a war is dependent on the ability to provide medical support to the troops (Captain Margaret Armstrong, United States Navy Nurse Corps, retired). Nurses have taken care of patients on and from the battlefield since the Crimea. Nurses were present in Vietnam in an advisory role early in the Vietnam era, as will be recounted by Kay Bauer in this book. The first hospital was opened by the United States Navy in 1962. Before the war was over, 5,283 nurses served for American forces. Eight nurses died during the war in Vietnam, one in action.

Nurses can do anything and they do everything. This is demonstrated by the personal accounts shared in this work. Common themes include reasons for joining the military, the desire to care for servicemen in a war time situation, love of country, concerns about the "rightness" or "wrongness" of the war, and discrimination against Vietnam veterans. They also talk about personal growth, times when they took responsibility for their actions and endured difficult situations, and opportunities for teaching and leading.

The Nurses at War Project

Since Florence Nightingale, Dorothea Dix, and Clara Barton, professional nurses have been involved in caring for the sick and wounded during military conflicts. This collection of accounts is of benefit to nurse-historians and others studying those who have served during military conflict. Collecting and archiving these accounts is critical because most of the nurses who served in World War I have died and nurses who served during World War II are now in their eighties, some with fading memory and declining health. Many voices are lost each day as this generation passes.

The Nurses at War Project is a continuing, long-term project to gather the accounts of nurses who have served during wartime. Accounts are gathered from nurses willing to tell their stories regardless of the war, the branch of military service, the site of service or the type of nursing performed. The main goal of the project is to acquire the accounts while the nurses are able to talk about their experiences.

Several common themes emerged as nurses discussed both their professional and personal experiences. First and foremost: "We did what we had to do." This is perhaps best exemplified in the words of an army nurse spoken with pride; who served during World War II "We had chosen a profession that required our best in brain and brawn." Professional themes included short staffing, long hours, and insufficient supplies calling for creativity and ingenuity in clinical practice.

Nurses treated victims of shock and trauma, as many of them practiced before the establishment of critical care units in the 1960s. They cared for patients with post-traumatic stress disorder (PTSD), which was not identified as an official diagnosis until after the Vietnam War. They cared for patients with unusual diseases not typically seen in clinical practice, including jungle rot and other skin conditions common in the Pacific theater in World War II. Sometimes they were in situations in which they were required to provide care beyond their scope of practice under very difficult circumstances. Often they had profound emotional experiences.

Some nurses made meaning of their war-time experiences, and described the lessons learned that profoundly affected their lives, including living fully in the present, reevaluating priorities, cherishing freedom, valuing home and family, and having faith and trust in God. These were the values they held fast to and which sustained them in difficult times. Nurses taking part in the project are very patriotic and speak of cherishing freedom, even in those instances in which they had conflicting feelings about going to war. Valuing home and family was a pervasive sentiment found in the interviews and in the letters written home. These nurses espoused a spiritual lifestyle, finding strength in their relationship with a higher power.

On November 11, 2004, Veterans Day, a note dedicated to nurses was left at the Vietnam Wall in Washington, D.C. It read: *"I don't remember your name, but thanks for saving my life."* This indication of how much the quiet, unsung, heroic services of a nurse meant to this veteran is inspiring. These men and women have made a difference in the lives of countless military personnel—and though they may not remember their names, they remember the reassuring presence and dedicated and competent care they received from a nurse.

Elizabeth R. Barker

Elizabeth R. Barker's story is one of developing leadership. Her leadership skills were clearly influenced by her experience in Vietnam, which influenced the rest of her nursing career. Her comments on the coping mechanisms of Vietnam veterans, both nursing and enlisted personnel, are important.

I always wanted to be a nurse. I can't remember ever wanting to be anything else. I was attending Wagner College on Staten Island in New York City. I didn't have money to continue college, so I went to see the Navy recruiter. I went into the Navy as a corpsman in April 1964, during Vietnam. They approved my continuing studies at Wagner in the Navy Nurse Corps Candidate Program. I graduated college in 1966 and went off to Newport, Rhode Island, as my first duty station. We did a lot of work with Vietnam casualties. We did a lot of training of the corpsmen to get them ready to go to Vietnam. We were training them how to pass NG tubes and start IVs and actually do tracheotomies, skills they might have to use when they got to Vietnam.

I had an instance one time where I was working the evening shift. I was going off duty through the emergency room. We had just received a good-sized group of casualties. They were on the deck and on stretchers. As I walked by, one of the casualties kind of tugged at my skirt. He had a tracheostomy and he put his finger in the trach and kind of rasped out, "Do you know Lieutenant Riley?" I said, "Yes, I'm Lieutenant Riley." "Do you know a guy named Henry?" I just rolled my eyes.

Henry was a corpsman we used to kid with a lot. We told him if we hooked him up with the Viet Cong we would probably win the war because he would screw them up so bad. This was a guy that just couldn't do things right. If you taught him how to do an IV, he had to do it 14 times to do it right. He would get all excited and couldn't figure it out. Like all the other corpsmen, he went off to Vietnam. The casualty said, "Henry said if I ever found you, I should tell you that you taught him to do it right."

Henry had performed a tracheostomy on this guy. Henry knew the patient would probably come back to the Newport area to recover because he was from the Newport area. They tried to put returning troops back in the region from which they came. It was really an amazing and wonderful thing to know the investment you had in time and energy to teach this corpsman something had paid off.

When teaching corpsmen how to put in IVs, they had to put one in us in order to pass off. Naturally, we had a lot of interesting puncture wounds on our arms. I was a very popular candidate because I have big veins. One night I was going across the parkway from the hospital to middle town, where I lived. It was kind of foggy, about 1930 (7:30 P.M.). There was a body lying across the road. I pulled over, stopped and jumped out of the car. It turned out to be some inebriated guy who had just passed out on the road. A police car went by and saw me leaning over this guy. The policeman stopped the car and got out to see what was wrong. I told him what had happened. Now, remember this was in the 60s and during Vietnam. This policeman saw my arms with all its band aids. He asked, "What happened to your arms?" I told him about teaching corpsmen to start IVs and practicing on us. He looked at me with a healthy grain of skepticism. I showed him my ID card and gave him my name. He said, "I think you'd better come with me."

He brought me back to the base and into the chief nurse's office. He wanted her to verify the fact I really was a Navy nurse, we really did let the corpsmen practice starting IVs on us and I was not a drug addict. I got a lot of teasing about that particular incident. I made sure I wore long sleeves afterward. Eventually we were able to roll the guy in the middle of road up on the berm. By that time he kind of woke up and walked off.

I was in Newport about two years. I tried to get orders to the submarine base in Groton, Connecticut. My husband was enlisted and stationed on a submarine. They never would acknowledge I was married and certainly were not going to transfer me to be with an enlisted man. I was married in 1966 to a man I met in college. He went into the Navy so he wouldn't get drafted.

I became pregnant in 1968. The rule was if you were a woman and had a dependent under 18 you couldn't stay in the military. We talk now about rights and privacy, but the reality was we really didn't have any privacy. We were in the Navy. When they gave you an order, you did it. I wasn't actually showing yet, so they figured they could get a couple more

6

months out of me. I had to go to the chief nurse and tell her I was pregnant. She looked at me absolutely dumbfounded. At that point if you were below lieutenant commander you were either addressed as "Miss" or "Mr." They never did want to change my name because I was married to an enlisted man and that was thought of as being terrible. She looked at me and said, "Miss Dawson, I just cannot believe you're pregnant." I said, "Yes, ma'am, I am." She said, "I don't know how that happened. We kept you on nights expressly to make sure this wouldn't happen." I found that pretty funny for her to think people who worked nights couldn't get pregnant. When my husband had liberty, he would drive up from Groton. It wasn't far. It was the big chuckle that I had sex other than in the dark of night.

My experience as a Navy nurse during that period was pretty intense. Those guys, who were mostly our age, were pretty badly hurt. There was a lot of intensive nursing at Newport with these fresh casualties. We had a lot of guys who had traumatic injuries and a lot of surgery. At that point, we didn't have very many antibiotics. We were just developing products like Betadine. It was very new. We didn't have any cephalosporins. The antibiotics we used were neomycin, tetracycline and penicillin; okay, but not great.

I worked in orthopedics. We would have guys with osteomyelitis because they had been wounded with punji sticks or had heavily contaminated wounds. They would have their leg surgically flayed open and have a neomycin drip going into their wound. They had a tube going into their leg with the neomycin running through it and another drain to suck out all the drainage. They were in horrible pain.

A lot of the guys came home having taken illegal drugs while they were in Vietnam. That was one of the ways some of them coped with being over there. They were debilitated by parasites and malaria and other conditions you get while you are in the tropics, in addition to their wounds. Postoperatively you would get an order for 75 or 100 mg of Demerol every four hours for pain control. These guys had been on a lot of drugs we didn't know about. They were withdrawing and we were giving them very small amounts of pain medication. Demerol and morphine were basically all the pain medications we had. These guys would be in terrible pain. We didn't know about or use things like morphine drips. The science of pain management simply did not exist yet. The doctors were very strict. If we actually gave pain medication every three hours, we were really setting ourselves up to go on report for overmedicating our patients. Everybody said, "We can't give them this pain medication because they will get addicted." What we didn't realize is they were already addicted.

We would spend tremendous numbers of hours with the patients, even during our time off. Your shift would be over and there would be guys you realized were just really in agony. We would go over and spend another six or eight hours holding their hand, talking and singing to them, and trying to keep their mind off it until they could have another pain shot. I wasn't the only one who did it. All the Navy nurses did it. We worked hard and we were very tired.

I know we were in the "safe zone." We didn't have to worry about rocket attacks and stuff like that, but we very seldom had a day off. On our days off we would come in to sit with the sailors, soldiers, and Marines to tide them over. The senior nurses weren't too happy about us doing that, but these guys really needed a lot of support. It was the only support we had to give them.

It was a very sad time because the way the public reacted to the war was to blame the military. They got angry with the politicians, but they also would get angry at the victims. They would be very abusive to those in the military and very abusive to these injured sailors and Marines.

I remember being angry at the injustice of the people who protested the war. I was angry at them for thinking those of us in the military, especially nurses and physicians, were people who thought it was okay to go to war. If you thought it was okay when you went in, having some strange perception war was glorious or noble, it didn't take you long to realize that was stupid. There isn't any glory in war, yet there were people who thought the people who were to blame for the war were the people in the military. That was the tragedy of that war. The members of the military didn't get support or acknowledgement. When it would come out that some were drug addicts, they were treated as criminals. These guys weren't criminals. They were trying to figure out how to cope with impossible situations and their response came out in very bad ways.

One time, at Newport, I went into the medication room. Another nurse was there. It didn't look like she was actually pulling up narcotics. When I asked her what she was doing, she said, "Just leave. Just get out of here." "No, what are you doing?" It turned out she was replacing Demerol with normal saline. She had a husband who had been a Marine in Vietnam and had come back horribly wounded. He decided he didn't want to live anymore. They had come to the conclusion she would help him commit suicide. She was going to take home enough narcotic so when he decided to kill himself she would have the narcotic ready for him. She told me this heart-wrenching story about this being the thing she could do for her husband and pleaded with me not to interfere. I understood she was doing what she thought was right. Her sense was her husband was the most important person in the world. She understood other people would have to suffer if she did this, but it came down to her being willing to do anything for her husband. He was a hero. I had to decide if I was going to be complicit or not. I made the decision I still think was the right, ethical decision. I reported it. She was gone within 24 hours and I have no idea what happened. The situation still causes me pain. I know she believed she was doing the right thing. I know I did the right thing. In doing the right thing there were a lot of people who were terribly hurt.

For those of us not in-country, that is in Vietnam, there is a lot of discussion about what our colleagues in-country experienced. They did go through amazing stuff. I can only imagine how awful that was. It was also not a picnic to be in CONUS, the continental United States, taking care of these guys. There were guys that would plead with you to let them die or plead with you not to let them die. You had no power one way or the other. You would just do the best you could. Some of the senior nurses would take us aside and tell us in no uncertain terms we had to be less involved. They wanted us to be less emotionally involved. I know that was the way they insulated themselves. It was a very traumatic time. I know I needed help to get through that.

I was fortunate in having a friend who knew of a French/American nun who was in Fall River, Massachusetts. She was a nurse existentialist. She was assigned to St. Anne's in Fall River, not too far from Newport. There were a couple of us that would talk to her. She taught us a lot about existential caring, how to be in I/thou relationships without destroying yourself, and how you learned to get as much from the relationship as you gave to it. You learned to be kind of like an artesian well, so you didn't go dry. You learned the danger signals. She was very helpful. She was one of the few people who never blamed the victim. She acknowledged what kind of a tough situation a lot of us were in.

One of the things that came out of the experience was I decided to go into OB as a specialist. I just wanted to get as far away from medical-surgical nursing as I could get. That is how I ended up as a clinical nurse specialist in high-risk perinatal (baby care).

I got out of the military when I became pregnant. I worked as a civilian nurse for a couple of years, then went back to school. Just as I was finishing my master's degree, the law was changed. Now they would let women be active duty with dependents. So, I went back in. The time I was civilian nurse was also a tough time. I think there were many military nurses who had the same experience. When we were in the military, we did a lot of independent stuff because we were the people that were there. When you got out into the civilian sector, you couldn't practice that way. You couldn't give the patient any information. You had to say, "You'll have to talk to your doctor about that," or "I can't tell you what your blood pressure is." You had to have permission to teach or to be a nurse. I got into trouble a lot. I think a lot of military nurses did. Some got out of nursing because of it.

———————————————————————

Elizabeth Barker retired from the Navy as a captain after working many years in women's health care. She continues to teach others to be outstanding nurses who are sensitive to the needs of patients, families and colleagues.

Catherine (Kay) M. Bauer

Catherine (Kay) M. Bauer tells of her experience in Vietnam as one of the nurses in-country during the early days of the war. She continues telling about serving in the United States during the Vietnam War, explaining the turmoil and unrest that existed then.

Kay struggled against poverty and prejudice to obtain her nursing education. Once in the profession she chose to serve in the United States Navy Nurse Corps and she served in numerous locations, performing many different types of nursing. She was about to resign her commission as an officer in the corps when she was offered the opportunity to perform a different type of nursing than she had ever done before—in a war zone in Vietnam.

I had requested an appointment with the Naval Hospital Director of Nursing (DON) Service to tell her my plans and resign my commission. She said, "Kay, just a minute. You have been in the Far East haven't you?" I had just come back from Japan and Guam. She said she had a position on a Navy surgical team headed to Vietnam with an OR nurse instructor and doctor who had been board certified as a general surgeon.

The DON called Washington as I sat there to get me assigned to this team. I would be a member of a seven-person forward surgical and advisory team. There were no U.S. military hospitals in the very south delta area of Vietnam. Thus, the Vietnamese would allow us to use one of their province hospitals in return for us providing surgical service to their military and civilian personnel as well as our own troops. We were also to be "advisors" to the Vietnamese nurses and the one doctor to help update their medical procedures.

I called home to tell my mom and dad I would be getting orders to Vietnam. My mom said to me, "Is Vietnam where you would like to go?" I said, "I think so." She said, "That's good." In the background I could hear my dad cussing a bit and saying. "There's a &%$+ war going on there!"

I knew there was a war going on. While in charge of pediatrics at

Great Lakes Naval Hospital, we taught basic pediatric nursing to the corpsmen sent to us from hospital corps school. Upon completion, they received orders to Fleet Marine Force School at Camp Pendleton, CA. From there they were sent to Vietnam with the Marines. They were like little brothers to us. If they had trouble with their girlfriends or wives or children, we would help them in whatever minor way we could. If they got married or had a child, we would have a small shower for them. We would listen intently as they told us of their plans for when they were finished with the Navy and asked our advice as to schools and training, etc. Then we started getting KIA/MIA (killed or missing in action) messages with the names of our corpsmen on them. That was very hard.

A week before we traveled to Vietnam, our entire team was sent to Washington D.C. to meet and be together before leaving the States. Our team consisted of an orthopedic surgeon, a senior ranking nurse, a second physician, a CRNA or nurse anesthetist, me, a Navy chief and a young Army captain medical service corps officer. His job was to speak "Army" for us. Other than a few advisors and the river patrol boats (RPBs), there was no Navy in our assigned area. All of our supplies would come via the Army. Our Navy chief, senior to me in age, was a very nice, talented man. He was both a laboratory and x-ray technician and had been in the Navy a while.

We were not on a military compound like the Army and Air Force nurses. The province hospital in Rach Gia, Kien Giang Province, in which we worked, was on the ocean at one side of the city. It had been built by the French shortly after the turn of the century. We had no running water or electricity and there were no screens on the louvered windows and doorways. We lived in a two-story house onto which some American contactors had added a second level. Our room was on that second level. It was so small we could barely walk around in it. The only bathroom was downstairs. The temperature outside hovered around and above 90 F. every day except during the monsoon, rainy, season when it dropped into the high 70s and low 80s. We wanted some space to walk around. We needed more room. Before long, we moved across the bridge from the hospital to another place. The United States Agency for International Development (USAID) could now send civilian nurses to work with us as there was room at our place for them. At times we attended USAID and joint US forces nurses' meetings in Can Tho, which was north of us at the US Army Fourth Corps Headquarters. South Vietnam had been divided by the Army into four headquarter areas: 1 Corps, 2 Corps, 3 Corps, and 4 Corps.

The Vietnamese had one doctor for five million people, but no surgeons. We provided surgery. Vietnamese patients couldn't see our doctors until they had been referred by the civilian doctor who was their chief of medicine. One day, Sergeant Phu, a sergeant with the ARVN (Army of the Republic of Vietnam), came to the other nurse and me. He was one of the smartest men I have ever met. When the Germans were there, he was sent to Germany to study medicine. When the French, Chinese, and Japanese were there, he was sent to their home universities to study medicine. He spoke all of those languages, including every dialect of Chinese, fluently. If we could not figure out via Vietnamese or English what a patient was attempting to say, we could talk with Phu. He would interpret for us. The Army assigned a medic to work with us and Phu. Some of them thought they knew much more than this Vietnamese sergeant. Finally, we were sent a really nice Army sergeant who was smart enough to know Phu was smarter than any of us and worked closely him.

We would go out into the areas around our city to see those who could not get into the hospital. We were careful not to venture out too far. One day Phu came to talk about the ARVN dependents. They couldn't be seen by the one civilian doctor because they were not civilians. They couldn't be seen by the one military doctor because they were not military. He asked if we would come over once a week and see them if he built a clinic. If we recommended the dependents be seen by either the civilian doctor or our surgeons, they could do so without anyone "losing face"! In about a week the clinic was built. We went there each week to conduct sick call. Many times we provided topical antibiotics, such as bacitracin ointment, or gave piperazine for intestinal worms, especially ascaris infestation.

Sergeant Phu asked if we would venture out into the deeper woods with his troops to get to some of those who were unable to get into the provincial hospital. He said not to worry because his heavily armed troops would go with us, and also everyone knew who we were and we cared for everyone. We were still a bit concerned until we actually saw the large number of "guides" decked out in various types of uniforms and an array of armament from head to toe!

In our home, we had an Army crank phone, such as you see on the movie *Mash*. We would be called from the hospital in the middle of the night when a bus or an area had been blown up. It was always at night when most of the action took place. At the hospital it was triage and treat. For any Americans involved, it also meant transport the next morning or asap. When we asked the number of Viet Cong personnel for whom we had provided care, after these events, we were usually told, "many," or, at times, "a few." The Vietnamese had very little medical care. They had a buddy system where they learned basic first aid to care for each other.

A U.S. Army advisor to an ARVN unit asked three of the nurses to go with him to an outer island one day. There had been an outbreak of plague and we were needed to administer the vaccine. We got permission from our commanding officer. Two of us said we would go. We were leery when we found out we were going via an Army boat. Our fears were soon realized.

Soon after the junk boat was finally underway, five hours later than the time we were told to report, the oil smell overcame so many aboard that most were vomiting. Fortunately, it was pouring rain so we went on deck and hovered under the tarps we had brought along. When we got out into, what seemed to us, the middle of the ocean, a smaller fishing boat came alongside. We transferred onto that, but it only took us to where we could see the island. We then rolled up our pants legs to wade the rest of the way into the beach. We carried our supplies of alcohol, glass syringes, steel needles, vaccine, a Bunsen burner, etc., on our heads and backs. This was before backpacks so we wrapped all of the supplies in our tarps and slung them over our shoulders or heads. All the nurses wore under our fatigues was swimsuits. We began giving the vaccine injections after doing some clinic work in a small tent the medics had set up.

As the hours passed and the sun was going down, I looked out and saw the boat from which we had waded into land, moving further out and around to the other side of the island. I walked over to the Army captain and asked where the boat was going. He said it was going to the leeward side of the island for the night. "How do we get back?" He said, "You are staying the night. Didn't I tell you?" I said, "No way! We only have swimsuits on underneath our fatigues, have nothing else along, and where do we sleep?" "We will stay at the mayor's house. However, before we do, we are expected to go to dinner at some of the councilmen's homes as soon as we are finished here."

Councilmen's homes were square huts made of bamboo fronds and pieces of salvaged tin with dirt floors and thin cloths hanging from the ceiling to divide the spaces into separate rooms. They cooked in the middle of the floor on kerosene stoves. We ate dinner squatting alongside them on the floor, then went to the mayor's house. The mayor had a house similar to ours in Rach Gia, with tile floors, louvered windows and doorways, but no electricity or running water. They had a separate, tiny, open-roofed building outside, housing a large cement tub of rain-water where we washed up a bit. We had shucked our fatigues and swam awhile to get clean when we realized our predicament. Swimming in our one-piece bathing suits was much to the dismay of the adult islanders. In their culture it was okay to be naked from the waist up, but very immodest to show off our bare legs! Now we just wanted to wash off the salt water. There was only one bedroom unutilized in the mayor's home. The nurses were not allowed to go in that bedroom as only the men were allowed there. Mosquito netting was draped from the ceiling around the large polished wooden table for us. In the morning they woke us so they could clear the table for breakfast for us and the family. We had a long talk with that Army captain when we returned to Rach Gia!

Another ARVN Army captain came to us at the hospital one day. He had received a portable generator and a new movie and wanted us to come and watch it with him and his men. We should have learned not to listen to Army captains, but we got in a jeep and drove over there after work. By this time, if a moving vehicle had a motor, we could figure out how to start it. We drove to the ARVN compound for the movie. We were so intent on watching the movie, we failed to note the time until we realized it was dark outside. We jumped into the jeep and took off for our abode. We knew the bunkers outside of the city on either side of the bridge were manned by armed troops at sundown. "I hope they realize this is our jeep coming in, because they have M–14s!" We drove over the bumps of that dirt road as fast as we could and made it home just in time to hear our crank Army phone ringing. The building in which we had been sitting had just been blown up by claymore mines the Viet Cong had set up while we were watching the movie! It was INSIDE of the ARVN compound! The whole area was blown away. If we hadn't left as soon as we did, we wouldn't be here today. Casualties from there, both Americans and the Vietnamese civilians and military, were brought into our hospital where we did triage and treatment the rest of the night. Several days later we went back to look at what was left of the structure and take pictures. One American and a number of Vietnamese soldiers had been killed.

We set up nursing education programs and taught those several times each week. Most of the Vietnamese nurses at that time had three months of training. Since there was only one doctor for five million people, nurse midwives handled all deliveries. Because of that, they were given about 18 months to 2 years of training. They were very good. Of course there was no such thing as a C-section, so those who needed one usually died, along with the baby they were carrying.

The hospital closed down at night. The families, who took care of patients all day, now enclosed the entire wards in mosquito netting and slept on the floors alongside the patients. A cement sluice ditch had been built many years before in the center of the hospital compound where water came in from the ocean, swirled through, and returned to the ocean. That water area functioned as a toilet, bathing area, laundry room, and a supplier of drinking and cooking water. Fresh water coming in was used for drinking, cooking, and washing clothes while bathing and then bathroom use was restricted to the area where the water swished back to the ocean. We had several large, cement cisterns collecting rainwater around the hospital that were used for drinking and cooking whenever it rained. Ocean water was only used when the cisterns were dry.

At our home, we had a large hole, about 5' × 7' in the ceiling of our "kitchen," beneath which was a huge, cement cistern, about the same size and 6 feet high. We finally commandeered some screening to put over that hole so nothing except water could drop into our cistern. We had little spigots on the sides of the cistern from which we could drain water for drinking and cooking. Every so often we could commandeer a portable generator to pipe water upstairs to our "bathroom" by a small spigot through which water could be forced to squirt onto us. It was cold, but at least it was running water to stand under.

One morning I awakened and pushed aside the mosquito netting around my wooden, four-poster, cot-type bed with wooden slats under a futon-type mattress. As I swung my legs over the side, my left leg felt very heavy. I looked at it, and saw it was twice the size of the other! I thought, "What on earth is going on?" Being bit by mosquitoes is something that occurred constantly of course. However, the day before, we had run out of gloves, so just washed our hands with alcohol between dressing changes. I was changing a dressing when a mosquito bit my ankle. I had just reached down and scratched it without thinking about it. I now had a red streak going from ankle to thigh!

I hobbled over to the hospital and the supply of penicillin was exhausted. We contacted our one Army pilot to ask him to fly to the various US and Vietnamese medical facilities around our area to find some penicillin. The only type in the field at that time was called Bicillin K, which was to be refrigerated. The pilot went everywhere. None of the US hospitals wanted to give any to him, especially when he told them it was for a Navy nurse working in a province hospital! Finally he did find some that was outdated by three years and had never been refrigerated. I gave myself shots with those long needles twice a day for about ten days. At least it took care of the infection so I did not have to be air evacuated to Saigon in either the one U.S. Air Force or the one U.S. Army two-seated plane in our city.

The day we arrived into Saigon, South Vietnam, we went to visit our friends at the Naval Hospital there. They were turning the hospital over to the U.S. Army that day. After that, we were the only two Navy female nurses in country during that year. This was 1966–67. The following year as we were leaving the country, the Navy started sending female nurses up north to Da Nang. I had gone there to visit at the request of the director of the Navy Nurse Corps who wanted a report on the hospital. As Florence Nightingale had written many years earlier, when only men run hospitals, there is a great deal of dirt! However, the doctors and corpsmen here provided treatment that was swift and wonderful!

The director of the Navy Nurse Corps asked if I would go on recruiting duty from Vietnam. I said I would go to Minneapolis. She said my friend was already there. Did I want San Francisco? No. New York? No way! Chicago? No. She asked where I did want to go. I said I would go to Quantico. That turned out to be really good for me. Since most of my patients were Marines who had just returned from Vietnam, I had an opportunity to sort through my feelings and some of my post-traumatic stress talking with them. I worked everywhere. I was in charge of our small, in-service education department while simultaneously working as head nurse, first on pediatrics and then SOQ.

Coming back to the U.S. from Vietnam, we were boarded on a civilian aircraft. We had been told to not wear our uniforms home so we were in civies before we landed. After landing at a California Air Force base, we stowed everything military into our bags then hailed a cab to the civilian airport. When I got aboard the Northwest Orient plane to Minnesota, there were several male and female flight attendants. One of the men asked if I had just come back from Vietnam. I was so surprised I stopped immediately and quickly scanned myself to see if I looked military, but could find nothing amiss. I was afraid to say yes, but worried about saying no. Finally, I told the truth. The attendant then said they had something special for me. Now I was really worried! But he smiled and asked if I would like a nice steak and some real ice cream. He showed me where I could lie down across the seats in the rear of the plane and brought extra blankets, pillows, and coffee. Wow! How different my homecoming was from so many of my friends. I eventually wrote to the airlines and told them about their wonderful attendants.

My chief nurse at Quantico called me in one day and said, "Check your schedule the day after tomorrow. I want you to get a fresh uniform and report to the White House." I was incredulous and said, "The White House?" "Yes, you have an invitation from the president to be there when he signs the bill allowing women in the military to attain the rank of general and admiral." A few days later I had lunch at the White House with Lyndon Johnson and Hubert Humphrey and about 20 other women from the Army, Navy, Air Force and Marine Corps. I know there were at least two or three Navy nurses there. President Johnson took pains to sign that bill with all 20 different pens so each of us could have one. That was an honor. The president talked to us and shook each of our hands as we were photographed. The photos were then sent to us at our duty stations. That was 1967. Until then, the only Navy female captain was the director of the Navy Nurse Corps, and commander was the highest rank any other female could attain. The same was true of the Army and the Air Force.

After Quantico, I was given the Minneapolis recruiter position. I recruited nurses from North and South Dakota, Minnesota, parts of Wisconsin, Iowa, Illinois and Michigan. On recruiting duty, I soon found no one outside of nursing understood what a nurse is or what kind of training is required to become a nurse. They thought we walked into a school, were handed a bedpan and a syringe, and presto, we were nurses. Even the commanding officers of the recruiting stations attempted to recruit men and women with inadequate backgrounds, telling them they would be given the necessary training in the Navy. Educating other recruiters as to requirements of nursing education, such as being a National League of Nursing (NLN) accredited school, etc., became a continuing additional duty.

I loved recruiting duty. I was privileged to work with the directors of schools and departments of nursing at all of the hospitals, colleges, and universities in seven states. This was the height of the Vietnam War. Male recruiters were being given a very hard time at those colleges and universities. I was often asked to go with them as they were not harassed as much when I was there. I would say to the protesters who besieged our display,

"Wait a minute. I just got back from Vietnam. Let me tell you what's going on here. If you don't like the war, don't talk to us. Talk to those who sign bills about war, your congressman and your representatives."

I always filled my quota so the recruiting command just kept increasing it! We are very blessed in the Midwest area with very patriotic citizens. In the 60s, we had many good schools, colleges and universities with nursing programs, and schools of nursing anesthesia. I recruited many nurse anesthetists. The critical shortage, as in every war, was for OR nurses and nurse anesthetists. If they were male, these nurses were usually sent to Vietnam. One man, a nurse anesthetist, came to me and said, "I'm going to join the Navy because I don't want to go to Vietnam, as my wife's pregnant. I know I am going to be drafted. I don't want to go in the Army. I want to go into the Navy. Promise me I won't go to Vietnam." I said, "I can't make you that promise." "Who can?" I said, "You can call Washington, but I doubt anyone can promise you that." He called Washington and they assured him he wouldn't go to Vietnam. He walked into my office about eight weeks later and said, "I was on my way to my duty station in Pensacola, Florida, with my wife and child when the state patrol stopped us to give me dispatch orders for Vietnam." His wife had already been to Florida and bought a home. He was irate. I said, "I cannot do a thing about it. I never promised you this would not happen." That was difficult.

I told those women who were being sent to Vietnam they would at least have access to running water and electricity, whereas I had not! My female Navy nurse recruits were not going to be sent to Vietnam. Most nurses knew to join the Army if they wanted to be sent to Vietnam immediately. The Navy usually wanted us to be in the military a few years before we were sent to an overseas duty station.

I had been on recruiting duty in my office in downtown Minneapolis for almost two years and was getting ready for work one morning. A call came from my Commanding Officer, "Kay, don't come into work today. Your office has been blown up." Eventually we learned some students from the University of Minnesota had been found. They had planted explosives to blow up the government building where my office had been as a protest to our involvement in Vietnam. My office was closest to the street and down a small flight of steps. On one side of the steps was my office. On the other side was a bathroom. It took a while to get it all repaired so I worked at the other end of the building.

I met and married my husband while I was in Minneapolis. We lived in a home just off a highway in St. Paul. It was not far from what, during World War II, had been an arms plant. During Vietnam, they were still making armaments for the military. Our home was on three acres of land, as was every home in that area. My office had one car we used when we were in town that had U.S. Navy recruiting signs on the sides. One of the chiefs, a lieutenant, and I took turns driving it, then picking up or dropping off the others. Thus, the Navy recruiting car was often parked in my driveway.

My friend came over one night to watch a Navy program on the television with me. Vern had gone to bed. The movie we wanted to watch started at ten o'clock. All of a sudden, we heard a terrible explosion. The whole house shook. I tried to dive under the bed. My friend ran outside to find out what happened. I was screaming, "Don't go outside, it's not safe!" By the time I got up off the floor and was running to the door, she ran back in and said to call the police and the fire department as the house next door was on fire. The fire department was already on their way. In the midst of this, my husband came out of the bedroom into the hallway and just missed being impaled by the roof entry door slamming down. The dent in the floor was three inches deep!

Someone had obtained plastic explosives from the arms plant and placed them behind the refrigerator of the house next door. The entire house just went up and came back down like a pancake and in pieces. It moved all of the rafters in our house. Pieces of their house were lying on top of our house, all over the yard and on the other side of the house as well. It was scattered around about nine acres of property. Our neighbors in that house had been asleep in bed and died in the explosion.

Suddenly two men I did not know were standing next to me on my lawn. It was not surprising to me as everyone within several miles had heard the explosion and were attempting to get as close to the action as possible, although the police and firemen had set up barriers. One of these men took my arm and pulled me aside to show his badge and ID card. He and the other man were from the Office of Naval Intelligence, now NCIS. He said I was to do two things now that both my office and the home next door had been blown up within the past months. First, I was to not drive a Navy car home again. How they knew I had been driving the Navy car I don't know, as it wasn't in my driveway at that time. Secondly, I was to find another house and move. The next day the headlines in the newspaper read, "Maybe They Got the Wrong House." That certainly did not make me feel very safe! Those who planted the explosives were never found. Eventually the neighbor's son built a new home on the site.

Later, my friend went back to active duty in the Navy. She had been back on active duty in North Carolina one week when I got a late evening call from a nurse who had been in Vietnam with me. I was excited to hear from her so started asking her many things. Finally, she almost shouted and said, "Kay, you'd better sit down. I've got something important to tell you. Please just sit down." She told me our friend had been out jogging around three o'clock in the afternoon, when she got off work, in the court-yard around the hospital at the Marine Corps base. Someone had come alongside her and said, "Can I jog with you?" She said, "Yes." All she remembers is that he was very young, perhaps, 18 or 19. The next thing she remembered was she was under a tree and he was punching her. He broke every bone in her face. Her face was wired for a long time and she later had to have abdominal surgery where his punches had damaged her internally so badly she had developed adhesions. She also had to have her spine fused. Of course, she was told it was her fault as she must have done something to cause that! She is medically retired from the Navy. ONI (NCIS) felt since she had been at my house the night when the house was blown up and now this happened there had to be a connection. While I am sure there were other such incidents in other places in the U.S., I haven't heard of them and do not know of any other nurse recruiters who had such problems. Terrorists do not think about what they are doing or whom they are damaging, only about their cause. How do they sleep at night?

Kay chose to leave active duty status in order to spend more time with family. She joined the Navy reserve and worked as a civilian nurse, working for the next 35 years in the same hospital. She went back to school for her master's degree. She and her husband were able to adopt a child and then went on to give birth to a child. Kay was active in the United States Navy Nurse Corps Reserve for 22 years. She remained active in advocating for patients and nurses. She was instrumental in beginning the Navy Nurse Corps session at the annual AMSUS (Association of Military Surgeons of the US) meetings. She was involved in the inception and formation of the Vietnam Women's Memorial in Washington, D.C., and formed support groups for nurse veterans, an idea that had its inception in Kay's Vietnam experience. Kay also served as adjunct faculty at a local college and a nurse educator in the community hospital setting.

Lou Ellen Bell

Lou Ellen Bell was an experienced United States Navy nurse when she went to Vietnam. Her story is a mature and detailed look at the Vietnam experience. The following are excerpts from that experience.

I was on recruiting duty when I received orders to Da Nang, Vietnam. I didn't have any qualms about going. I wanted to go. I asked to go. Whenever I asked to go, the Navy detailer said, "How many more recruiters am I going to have ask to go?" I guess we were all requesting that as our next duty station. It was hard to talk about the need for nurses in combat when you hadn't been there. I ended up with some of the people I knew, though none of those I recruited. The Navy wasn't sending them over quickly, which was a good thing. The Army nurse that was recruiting was fresh out of a college baccalaureate (BS) program. She spent six months at Fort Bragg, and they sent her to Vietnam. I cannot imagine, with such little nursing experience beyond a BS degree, being able to cope with the situation in Vietnam.

When we arrived in Vietnam, we called for someone to come get us, as per our orders. We were supposed to call the chief nurse. They wouldn't put my call through to the chief nurse because it was after bedtime. I told them who I was and why I was calling and they still were refusing. I said, "Well, let me speak to the officer on duty." I spoke to him and he assured me he could not put a call through to the nurse's quarters. I said, "Well, there are five Navy nurses over at the terminal. Would you arrange to have transportation come pick us up and take us to the hospital?" He said, "Oh, certainly." He called main administration and asked them to send someone. They said they didn't have anyone. Ultimately the transportation came from the hospital.

I told the officer of the day there were five women and a whole lot of luggage. Each one of us had two and three pieces or more. I told him to make sure they brought something big enough to hold everything. The truck that came was a pickup with a cab large enough for the driver and five passengers. The back was closed in so people could sit there or it could be used for cargo. As it pulled in, we headed out to it and saw doctors getting into our cab. They were, of course, in long pants and we were in dresses, our light blue uniforms. It was very hard, in a dress, to get up in the back of a truck. The driver, bless his little heart, was a young enlisted man. He said, "Excuse me sirs, I came over here to pick up five nurses and five nurses will be in the cab before this truck will move. If you care to come with us, you can get in the back." He called and got another truck to pick up our luggage.

As we were on our way to the hospital from the airport, you couldn't go beyond a certain point without showing identification. It was not American military personnel at those checkpoints. They were Vietnamese. They were the Vietnamese we were there to support. When you approached the concertina wire, like barbed wire, at these checkpoints, the only way you could get past was to get clearance through this person who was a foreign national.

We didn't go directly to the hospital. We went to something called the "White Elephant," which were the administration offices for the whole area. We had to fill out a lot of papers. I said, "Is there a possibility we could finish this tomorrow? We are very tired. I don't know about anybody else, but I'm not thinking clearly enough to fill out all this paperwork." He said, "Well, I don't know. You really need to finish this paperwork." I said, "That's fine, we will do it tomorrow. Please take us home to the hospital." When we got there, the chief nurse had heard we were coming. A lot of nurses were up to greet us. We got to bed about four o'clock in the morning. This young MSC officer had told us we needed to be up and ready at eight A.M. to go finish checking in, which we did. By eleven or so we had done all kinds of stuff.

It was so hot, at least 120 degrees. It was July in Vietnam. I said to another nurse checking in the same time I did, "I'm about to pass out." She echoed the exhaustion. I said to the MSC officer, "Is there some place around here that is cool that we can get something cool to drink?" He said, "No, the only place would be back at the hospital." I said, "Good, so take us back to the hospital so we can have lunch." He said, "You need to finish checking in." I said, "I'm not doing anything else until we have a chance to get something cool to drink and an opportunity to find out who we are again. We're exhausted." Nobody contested. There was nobody really senior to me. I think somebody else was a lieutenant or lieutenant commander, which is the same as I was. I had just come from recruiting and so I was

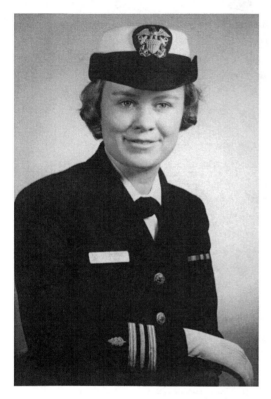

pretty bossy. He said, "Well, I'll pick you up at one o'clock and we'll go finish checking in." I went to get something to eat. I figured I'd be all ready if I did that. The others went to their quarters. They had just had all they could endure. That may have been also why they weren't talking. When they got over there, Mary Cannon took one look at them and said, "Go to bed. You're not worth anything to me until you get some rest." When I got over there, she told me the same thing. She said, "Right now if I needed a nurse on duty there is not one of you that could work." I said, "But he told us we needed to finish checking in." She said, "And you can do that tomorrow. I'll take care of it."

Mary Cannon was the chief

Lieutenant Commander Lou Ellen Bell.

nurse that was leaving. Helen Brooks came after her. Mary Cannon was an Army nurse for several years. She had gotten out of the Army and come into the Navy. She was the first chief nurse in Vietnam with a large contingency of nurses. They opened the hospital there.

The accommodations there were pretty decent. They had taken Quonset huts and divided each into eight units. You walked through the front door into a narrow hallway with four small rooms on each side. My bed was five feet long. In order to turn it across the room I had to disassemble it and reassemble it. I think the room was about six feet wide and about eight feet long. It had a sink in it. Bathrooms were out of the hut and down a covered sidewalk which was our hallway. There were four showers, but the Seabees had made a stainless steel tub out of one of them. They made the tub six feet long and four feet wide. We were on water rations and so nobody could use it. If you put an inch of water in it, you would have used all the water you would have used for a shower. I used it one time and I was embarrassed I had used that much water. The room with the four showers in it and the adjacent room had a deep sink and a washer and dryer. After I got there I managed to persuade the chief nurse to get a refrigerator in there so we could have a beer mess. In the little room there was a bank of sinks. There were four or five commodes, each one partitioned off with a door. Each of the huts, except the bathroom, was air conditioned. The shower was ventilated but not air conditioned. Our only phone, a hospital phone, was in the passageway.

There were four huts for the females. These were all on the four corners if you can imagine an *H*. Off the middle of the *H* on the one side was the shower in the bathroom-type facility. In the opposite direction was the third hut and that was our little community gathering space plus the chief nurse and the assistant chief nurse's room. There were three rooms there but the big one was supposed to be the chief nurse's room. She elected to move to the side and saved the big one for a small living room we used for guests whenever they came. The director of the Navy Nurse Corps, Captain Bulshefski, used that room when she visited. Usually they had a three-room apartment there with their own bath in it.

When I was on nights sometimes, Helen Brooks would ask me to come over and wake her up. I'd step into that area just to wake her up. When Captain Bulshefski was leaving, I brought over some sweet rolls by Helen's request and woke Helen up to tell her the admiral was leaving. The other nurses would join them in the lounge and say their goodbyes.

When I first got there, we had Vietnamese girls clean our quarters. They did a so-so job. One day I went in and one of them was washing somebody else's shoes under running water. I persuaded Helen to request a steward to be assigned to our quarters. I had done a little homework figuring out how many people were giving up their housing allowance to live there. Other than the people who had dependents, which most of us didn't, there was a lot of money there. Since the military was saving money and providing minimal quarters I thought they could provide a steward to make sure the quarters were maintained. She looked at that and thought it was a good idea. She took it to the commanding officer and we ended up with a steward.

There was the idea a man couldn't be assigned to women's quarters.

That was her first objection. I said, "Why not? There are workmen in here all the time. None of us come out without being dressed, at least with a robe on." We never knew if we were going to find a guy in our little hut's passageway changing a light bulb or painting. I said, "So that's not the problem. They can be out here and they can knock on somebody's door before going into a room. If somebody was in their room sleeping, the door will be closed with a sign on it to not disturb."

Before having a steward, a nurse was left in our quarters during the day to supervise the Vietnamese women. We weren't worried about them stealing anything. We had lockers in our rooms. They just needed education on how to take care of things. Their standards of what to do were not the same as ours. It was a constant struggle to get them to sweep, mop, and clean the sinks and bathtub. The steward was a Filipino first class petty officer. The doctors had all kinds of stewards over at their place. I thought they could spare one. We deserved some of that care. Then the steward could have on his resume that he supervised five Vietnamese nationals. He was very nice and a little embarrassed when he first came but then he took charge. If there was maintenance work to be done, he would be there when the maintenance guy came rather than somebody on our staff having to be there.

We had about six or eight nurse anesthetists. Their quarters were separate though they connected with ours. The space in between contained a few beds. It was where they had put us when we first got there. We actually had just bed space. We had to come into the main quarters to go to the bathroom. Unless there was a vacant room because somebody had gone or somebody was out on leave, that's where nurses stayed overnight waiting for the hospital ships. It was not air conditioned. It was air cooled when the wind blew.

Margaret Higgins, one of our nurses, had decided to get garbage cans and put them underneath each of the air conditioning units to collect the water. Then she used the water to raise her farm. We called it Higgie's Farm. It was a small area of sand between two of the huts. She had someone send her seeds and she planted vegetables.

The Seabees built us a charcoal grill. They made it so tall we ultimately ended up digging a hole to put it down lower to the ground so we could reach it. Initially, we had to pull a stool up so we could reach the grill. If you want anything done by the Seabees, just know it's going to be grandiose. We had picnic tables there and that is where we could entertain. We

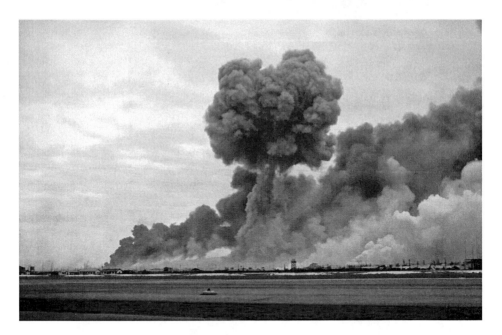

Incoming rockets.

couldn't entertain in the building. We also had a banana tree, which could have been there compliments of Higgins. That was our social gathering place. Individual dating was usually done at the officer's club.

Incoming rockets were usually not too bad. One night I was at MAG 16, our Marine Air Group across the street from where we were. There were several of us there and we got incoming hitting the sergeant's club. I called the chief nurse as soon as I got a chance to let her know I could see the area where the nurses were and I knew that area was not hit. She told me to get them together and bring them back as soon as possible. I said, "I'm sorry. I can't do that right now. This base is on lockdown and we can't get off of it at the present time, but as soon as we can, we'll come home."

When we first got there, we were working eight-hour shifts. I was in orthopedics. A lot of the American military would come in at night and would leave by noon the next day on their way home. When they were first in Vietnam, they were bringing them directly back to stateside hospitals. Then, they found out it was not good for the patients to travel so far and so long, so they slowed the process down. Most of our patients were going

27

to Japan and other areas. The Air Force was doing the transport. Most of the patients were sent to the Air Force facility to stay overnight and fly out the next morning. The flight nurse would come to the hospital and get a direct report from the night nurse. The patients would be loaded and taken directly to the plane. They were called "Arrive and Fly." They arrived at the airport and flew out immediately.

The other end of the orthopedic ward was other nationals, including POWs that were too sick to be over on the POW ward. They would be on whatever ward they required for care. They would require a Marine guard to sit with them for their protection. Usually they would be too sick to be a threat to anybody else but it was a two-way thing. The Marine was there for the protection of the prisoner. I had one North Vietnamese woman wake up to find she had no leg on one side. She probably blamed all of us. Our communications were between "nil and none." She reached out and grabbed my arm and just about pinched a hunk out of it. I was trying to do something to help her. We also had Korean nationals, Vietnamese and Montagnards. The Montagnards were an organized fighting force. I heard they were very good fighters.

When there was a military person injured in the field, his unit would call for a helicopter. They would say the nature of the injuries. They could be directed to the Army, Navy, or one of the hospital ships; wherever they felt they could best get care. For example, if the patient had an eye injury and our ophthalmologist was gone for some reason, then they would redirect the helicopter to the hospital ship. The easiest thing for us to do was to work with the hospital ship. There is something to be said for coordination.

Normally there would be only one hospital ship close to us at a time. They would alternate. One would go north while the other one went south. One would go up closer to the DMZ and then they would come down to our area. When an injured patient arrived at our place, they went into receiving. They had "Receiving 1" and "Receiving 2." Generally, the injured came by helicopter. When the helicopters would call in ahead of time, the stretcher bearers ran out to meet them with folded stretchers. For each patient received on a stretcher, they would give a folded stretcher to the helicopter crews to use for the next patient. The stretcher bearers were primarily nonrated enlisted men, not corpsmen. People that were not corpsmen were sent to the hospital to work. They would assign them to push food carts up to the ward for about three months to build up their muscles.

On ship they might chip paint but here they were pushing chow carts to the wards. The stretcher bearers came from that pool. You'd have to be strong to carry those patients. They had to run from where the plane landed to the receiving area. Most of the patients went to "Receiving 1," which was an open-bay area. There were sawhorses already set up where stretchers could be placed.

IVs were also set up with the IV sets attached and ready to place. I don't know how long they were kept before being broken down. These IV's hung all over the place. There were poles attached to the length of the wall or overhead and the IV's were hung by "S" hooks to the poles. We still had glass bottles in Vietnam. They started IV fluids in plastic bags but I think they went to the field corpsmen. Glass bottles would be dangerous and hard to carry in the field. The advantage of the plastic was you could start it and then stick it underneath the patient's shoulders. The pressure from their shoulder would push the fluids in.

"Receiving 1" saw the bulk of the patients. There was a cover but the outside temperature was the room temperature. "Receiving 2" is where the worst injured patients were treated. The capacity was eight patients. The patients were seen and immediate care was given in an air conditioned, cleaner environment with considerable emergency equipment. From the receiving areas, patients were assessed, stabilized and identified, and decisions made as to the surgery required.

The first piece of identification the patient received was the blood number. The blood number was written with a felt-tipped pen on their chest. Blood was drawn and sent to the lab. That number was matched to whatever their blood number ID was. In an emergency sometimes you are treating a patient before you know who they are. One senior corpsman had the job, in the receiving area, to go through patient clothes and secure valuables. He determined the person's identity and put everything in a bag. They would put armbands on the patients as soon as they were able to and then get them admitted. In the meantime that blood number was the way of identifying each of them, their records, personal belongings and lab samples.

From there the most immediate adjacent facility was up the sidewalk. On the left was the x-ray department and on the right was the pre-op for the OR. Before the patient left our receiving they would usually slip them onto what they called hardboard. This is a piece of plywood on stretcher rails with a sheet over it. The wooden hardboard could be put directly onto the x-ray table and eliminated the need to move the patient on and off the x-ray table as x-rays could be done through the patient and the board.

From there the patients went to pre-op. The patients were held in pre-op until they could go into the OR. We had two major operating rooms. They were in a framed building with linoleum on the walls so the walls could be washed. The floor was covered with small tiles. I noticed the OR table had managed to chew up a couple of tiles. I looked at the walls to see how much of it was washable. There was linoleum up about four or five feet. They had hanging overhead lights and metal cabinets. It was pretty neat for a war zone.

I saw the other ORs were Quonset huts. The two operating rooms in the Quonset huts were back to back with a dividing half wall in between the operating tables. The rooms were open on the sides so you could walk from one operating room to the other.

They also had a mash unit which was the back of a truck. Something they could just set off and set down, a metal box type thing. One was a dental OR. It was prefabricated out of metal and could be loaded onto the back of a plane.

When the female nurses first arrived they found urinals in the operating rooms for the medical staff to use in between surgeries. I never saw them. I only heard about it. It speaks to the massive numbers of surgeries the staff were handling in those operating rooms prior to the construction of the new operating rooms. These units continued to be used as needed on a daily basis.

Most of our wards were Quonset huts. At one time I had a Vietnamese female that was diagnosed with typhoid. We had a couple of individual rooms in some of the Quonset hut wards and she was put in one of those on isolation.

When you think about being out there in that kind of heat and wet and bacteria with the rashes and then you get infection, you've got a mess. Our chief nurse, Helen Brooks, had been in Korea and was very smart about this. She had shipped this huge box of socks to herself in Vietnam. Anytime one of the corpsmen who had worked with her came by to say "hi," she always gave them a few pair of socks to take back to the field with them. When she was in Korea, she found that the men in that theater of war never had enough socks.

Prior to leaving for Vietnam, I talked to someone who had been there. They told me to have extra soles put on the bottom of my shoes because of the unevenness and the rocks. I took brand new shoes and put new soles over the existing sole. It made all the difference in the world in terms of comfort. The other thing that she suggested was I buy cotton underwear because cotton absorbs perspiration.

After the patients had their surgery and went through recovery, they'd go to ICU if they were critical. When I say "critical," I remember the night I stopped by there and heard somebody saying, "I don't know why that patient is here? They only have this and this. I don't know why they're in ICU." I said, "I know you guys are accustomed to all this, but may I just point out this person has a head wound, a chest wound, a belly wound and would be in ICU in any stateside hospital." I had worked on the surgical unit, and I knew they had patients that were very sick in the surgical unit. They all just thought that was the biggest laugh. They had all been there so long and their patients were so critical that they had kind of gotten accustomed to a little less ill patients being considered not as critical and not sent to ICU.

ICU was staffed well with nurses because they needed a higher patient-nurse ratio. The rest of the place had one nurse covering more than one ward. Some of the younger nurses worked in ICU as well. The other place that some of the younger nurses worked was the surgical unit. One side was general surgery and the other side was neurosurgery.

One time I was on the night shift. I had a neurosurgery patient come back from the OR without an order for an antibiotic or a steroid. I called the doctor, and that's something we didn't do because they got precious little sleep. When he came to the phone, I told him what it was and he said, "I'll be right there." I said, "Well sir, you don't really need to come over. I just wanted to know if you intentionally didn't write for an antibiotic and a steroid." He came over and wrote the order and said, "I just wanted to meet the nurse that knew there should be an order and had the guts to call me." He also wanted to know why I wasn't assigned to neurosurgery. I told him that I also had orthopedics experience and I usually worked there.

Another person I thought was wonderful was Walt Godfrey, an MSC officer. He came over as our supply officer. One of his responsibilities was restocking all of our supplies. He set up automatic restocking almost as soon as he got there. It was a little bit of a hassle at first because we had to decide how much of each item we wanted on the shelf at all times. The items and number were put on the shelves and restocked daily. This was better than handwriting a stock order every week or two. Also, stocks of supplies didn't pile up in one area needed in another area. From the time Walt came, supplies were not my problem. Maybe the general idea of an automatic stocking system came out of the war.

While I was in Vietnam, a patient came in with a live grenade in his eye. They brought him in with a flak jacket over his head. They wanted somebody to stabilize his head. The corpsman that did it later told me without even thinking, he had voluntarily held the man's head. He was holding the patient's head as they moved the patient to the OR. Then he realized that this grenade could go off at any moment and his hands were under the flak jacket. The only thing to do was to get it out as soon as possible. They called the explosives group to stand by. The OR staff were all volunteers. They took him into the OR and the doctor was able to get it out without it going off. They gave it to the bomb squad and they disposed of it. I know the whole crew got awards for bravery. Most importantly, the patient survived.

I was a lieutenant commander and 33 years old in Vietnam. I had been in the Navy Nurse Corps for over 12 years. I wanted to go to Vietnam because I came in the military to be a military nurse. I had a lot of experience and I felt the patients were entitled to some of that. Most of the nurses I worked with were experienced. The majority of them were lieutenant commanders with some lieutenants. We didn't have an ensign on our staff and we only had one Lieutenant JG that I remember at Naval Station (NSA) Da Nang while I was there.

The corpsmen said I didn't check all their IVs every night every hour or two. They said that when I checked one, it was always one that had failed. One of the younger nurses asked how I did that. I said, "I don't really know. One might have a sixth sense something might be wrong. I think it is just experience." I think maybe I would look at them but not necessarily walk over to them. As I talked with the patient I would look at the drip of the solution but I didn't stand there and count it. I expected them to check the IVs and bring it to my attention.

We were near the beach but we didn't have the opportunity to go often. You couldn't walk anywhere other than on the hospital compound. There was a small exchange and a few places to eat. There was a place to get our uniform laundry done or pay the Vietnamese to do it. It was a rather self-contained hospital compound. If you wanted to go to the main exchange, you had to call for transportation. Normally they liked you to

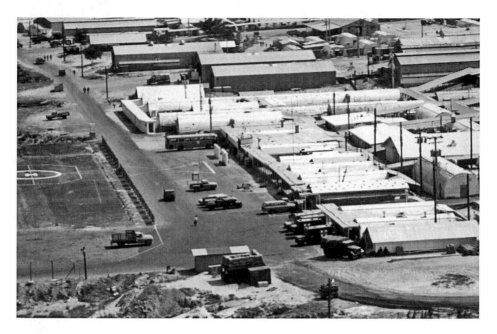

NSA Hospital, Da Nang.

get a group together. At China Beach, named for the China Sea, there was an exchange. You wouldn't go down there by yourself. I didn't like to go to China Beach because that's where all the troops were. MAG 16 had a private beach across the street and I enjoyed the privacy. That whole strip along there was beach. The Marine airstrip was between us and the water. We were not far from it but you couldn't walk there from a safety stand point. We never left our compound, even to go to the beach without some-one to drive us. At our command, the females were not permitted to drive. When I questioned the chief nurse about this, she replied that I would need a government driving license. I had one. Then she said that I would need to know how to shoot a weapon, and I told her that I had been on a pistol team at a previous duty station. Her final reply was, "How would it look?" I concurred that we might be viewed as easy targets.

After Nixon came into office the amount of casualties dropped. He apparently told the military we could only take a defensive stand. The patient load lightened up a bit. I got a chance one day to go up to Quang Tri. I wanted to see the hospital. We rode up on a Jolly Green Giant, which was an Air Force helicopter. We flew up to Quang Tri and then they took

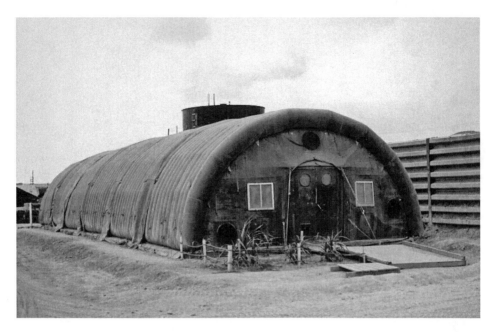

Inflated ward, 3rd Marine Division Hospital, Quang Tri.

us by jeep over to the hospital. The only nurses there were the male nurse anesthetists. I met the head nurse of ICU, which was a corpsman. One interesting thing about this hospital was they had some inflatable wards. It resembled the curved shape of the Quonset hut, but the walls were supported by inflatable chambers in the walls.

The corpsman that was in Quang Tri ICU took advantage of the fact he had nurses there and asked their opinions. He did a consultation about some of his patients and asked for suggestions. That must have been quite a stress to have that much responsibility. I think he was a corpsman that had gone to "C" school. It is a year and a half advanced training. These guys can be sent on a ship and be the chief medical officer for the ship. These men could probably come home and take the OPN (LPN) boards or go into the PA program. A lot of the earlier PAs were ex-corpsmen.

Two of the four nurses who traveled that day to Quang Tri left on the air evac plane that took patients to Da Nang. We found later that they were unable to land in Da Nang because the ammunition dump was exploding. Val Pack and I remained in Quang Tri to return later with the same Jolly Green Giant helicopter. We were offered an opportunity to go to

Dong Ha, a smaller medical facility about 6 miles from the DMZ. Travel was via jeep. This facility treated a lot of children. We did not remain long, then returned to Quang Tri, only to be told that we probably could not return to Da Nang that day because of the explosions at the ammo dump. This was the first we had heard about it. Finally, we got the chaplain to take us to the airport to see if the Jolly Green was returning and it was. So we boarded the plane and returned.

Just as we got off the chopper, a pickup truck came out and picked us up. I got into the truck and decided to take a picture of an explosion as it was happening. The pickup driver said, "Put your fingers in your ears and open your mouth." I said, "Huh" and he said, "Huh, hell! Just do it!" Immediately following the plume from the explosion would be a concussion wave. If you didn't plug your ears, the concussion wave would rupture your eardrums. It was something that had to be done immediately. The minute that it took passed. The corpsman took his fingers out and so did I. He said, "Ma'am, I'm sorry but you had about a second to get your fingers in your ears or you were going to have permanent ear damage." I thanked him for alerting me any way he could.

I was in Vietnam from July 1968 to July 1969.

The nurse who had been my recruiter, who had been a flight nurse during World War II, told me that the Navy nurses were extremely protected versus the Army nurses. The Army nurse wore fatigues. The Navy nurses came in a dress uniform. She said she remembered one time, and I don't know where she was, she asked for a bucket so she could wash her hair. The guy said, "Use your helmet like everybody else." She said, "I don't have a helmet. I'm a Navy nurse." " Oh, I am sorry ma'am. I'll get you a bucket." Navy nurses were treated differently because of how they dressed, no helmet and a dress for a uniform. I thought wearing whites on duty in a war zone was the stupidest thing I'd ever heard of. But, Mary Cannon, the previous chief nurse had been an Army nurse and she told me she wasn't going to be the Navy nurse that put Navy nurses in fatigues. The hospital laundry had to launder our uniforms so that they were washed, pressed, and starched. We had one washer and dryer in the quarters, but that was for other personal items.

A Vietnam woman had been raped on the hospital compound. So, we had to be escorted by a Marine escort, especially at night, wherever we went unless we were on the ward. I think I had the only ward assignment where you had to walk outside to other wards that I covered. There was just an uncovered sidewalk through some areas that were support buildings and not occupied at night. It hadn't been worrying me at all until this incident. So, if I could, I would get a corpsman to walk with me. Otherwise I had to get a Marine guard to come to escort me.

So, I had this corpsman walking along with me. He was in his fatigues with his flak jacket on. I am walking in my white uniform with my white cap and my white hose and white shoes. We were walking in an area where we could be seen from the fence line. Beyond the fence line was no man's land. He said, "Excuse me ma'am. I don't mean any disrespect, but would you mind walking further ahead of me? I don't know if you realize what a great target you are." "Oh yes, I realized that right along. But look at it this way. If Charlie hits me, he will be darned sure he hit a nurse. It is probably going to be the last of him and everybody else in the area." He said he wasn't sure that would protect him. But I had been walking through this area ever since I had been there and nobody had even taken a shot at me. We also had Marines in towers in raised pillboxes on the perimeter of the hospital compound. The hospital compound was an entity unto itself. It wasn't part of a larger compound. It was a relatively small compound. I felt pretty protected. But, I never had to test that theory. The only concern was incoming mortars and even when that happened they would say, "Oh they were just short rounds. They were aiming for MAG–16 across the street."

The following are excerpts from letters to my mother during that time.

25 January 1969—I had been to Hong Kong and back. I did tapes as well. I did letters only when I was on duty. I said, "You know, turn a woman who hasn't been shopping in six months loose in the greatest shopping center in the world and watch out. Seriously, I had a ball and it was worth every cent of it. The greatest treat of all was talking to my family." I had just told my mother about all these things I had bought. I bought shoes and had a coat handmade and a camera. Some of this I just had shipped straight home. Some of it I brought back to Da Nang and shipped it out from there when I came home.

4 February 1969—This was my pay entry base date. "Dear Mom, do you remember what we were doing twelve years ago today? We drove up to Raleigh, North Carolina, and I was sworn into the Navy Nurse Corps. I never knew then I would still be in twelve years later. A lot has happened in those years, hasn't it? I've been to Portsmouth, Cuba, Charleston, Boston, Philadelphia, Pittsburgh and now Vietnam. I've gained experience

I would never have had if I had stayed at James Walker." James Walker
was my nursing school. "Not to mention getting my BS degree (while I
have been in the Navy). There have been some good years and some bad
ones. Sometimes I wonder what our life would have been like if I had not
left Wilmington."

"Occasionally I think seriously about getting out of the Navy. But you
know how much I'm part of that and it's a part of me. That's where my
friends are and so I'm a lifer,' as they say, here in Da Nang. I can still think
of getting out if I should find a prince charming, though it does seem likely
he has been found by somebody else."

"I have some news for you. I got a real surprise today. It wouldn't come
as a surprise to you. As you would say, I knew that you would get it,' but
I really wasn't expecting it. When I got up tonight at 18:00, I had a letter
under my door. I have been accepted for school in rehabilitative nursing.
There is just one problem and it makes me view this with mixed emotion.
I'm going to go to the State University of New York in Buffalo. (My family
lived in Florida). I'm convinced they're trying to make a Yankee out of me.
I will be going in September and I will be able to take a four month leave
and maybe even assigned TAD somewhere for a couple of weeks, hopefully
near home. I don't know what to say. I have been somewhat depressed at
the thought of being so far from home again and in the cold weather. I
know it's a lot closer than I am now. I should be very pleased they think
I'm worth sending to school."

4 February 1969—"Naturally there's a lot to do so I'm just now taking
a break. I only have two active orthopedic wards. On one ward they admitted seven patients today and one we received tonight. On another ward
they admitted seventeen patients today. They discharged fifteen; those
were going out air evac to Japan. We also transferred nine up to a third
ward, a convalescent ward. I was just drawing some blood for crossmatch
on two POW patients that will have surgery in the morning. I am, at the
same time, starting an IV so we will have the needle in the vein to give
blood for their surgery. I must run now. I have to check on my patients
and go to midnight chow." This was really all before midnight or 1:00 am.
I worked from seven at night until seven in the morning. I added four more
patients on my ward between 7:30 P.M. and midnight.

We were mostly dependent on eating in the hospital with an occasional
meal at the officer's club. We had a small refrigerator in our quarters, but
it wasn't big enough to put much in with a bunch of us eating.

23 February 1969—"Just a note to let you know I'm safe, sound and happy. I heard on the news today Da Nang is under attack with many casualties. I guess that story is even bigger back at home. Fact is they managed to hit an ammunition dump about four miles away at the deep water piers and, I think, the airport. We did receive many patients but nothing worse than last August. We do anticipate more activity. However, everybody is on guard. I don't think we have anything to worry about except receiving casualties, so don't you fret."

26 February 1969—"Just another short note to let you know things are not so bad here. I get scared every time I listen to the news. More so than what is actually happening. The Da Nang Air Base and the Republic of Vietnam storage area were attacked. That was several days ago but thus far things have been exceedingly quiet here. We've been on alert several times but they haven't even hit MAG 16, across the street. Most everything has been in town or at Freedom Hill." I didn't tell her that Freedom Hill wasn't that far away." They hit the Navy Exchange storage area over there, which means they got the booze. They really didn't get it but they destroyed it. You should have heard the moans about that. But Mom, they are really hitting some of our boys in other areas. We've been receiving quite a few but it isn't any worse than I've seen before. We seem to be under a little more pressure, as I know everybody is concerned that this is the start of another offensive like last year's attack. Actually the intelligence reports are that they had been able to prevent them from having the ability to strike like they did last year. Please remember we are probably very safe here. The Marines guard this place well and I'm not just saying this to make you feel better."

14 March 1969—She had asked me about picking up something at the Navy Exchange and I couldn't. I said, "I'd like to do that but I have a ration card for all of this year. The only way I could get it would be if I could get out of country on leave. We are permitted one refrigerator, one TV, one regular camera, one movie camera, one slide projector, one movie projector and a couple of watches. Otherwise the small amount that does make it into the country would be purchased by the people who have the time to go to the exchange regularly. Right now all they have in stock are cassette recorders."

"The only real opportunity for much buying is on R&R or leave. We only had four days in Hong Kong. We arrived about 23:30 Sunday night and left about 06:00 Friday morning. Actually I feel like I did pretty well for the time I was there. You may have heard we had some excitement here. It seems a Chinese Communist mortar fell in an open field between the cook's quarters and ward 5B. As it happens, a few people picked up some slight flesh wounds. Both places were practically deserted as most everybody was at the movies. This incident could have been a real disaster. The patients and the corpsmen attend an outdoor movie in the middle of the compound. Had the mortar landed about fifty yards from where it did, it could have done some real damage to approximately 200 people. It was the first incident of war damage and personnel injury on our hospital compound since I've got here. It was fortunately very mild. Everybody here said that it must have been amateur night as it was the only mortar received anywhere around in the whole area. Hitting a hospital is a 'no no.' The American press eats it up. I hope you haven't been too worried. I was safely in my quarters at the time. I missed all the excitement." I didn't tell her how close my quarters were.

20 March 1969—"The hospital got hit again earlier tonight. Fortunately there was not one casualty, not even a scratch. It hit just the entrance to a ward sending shrapnel into the ward. It scattered more around the area. I repeat, no injuries whatsoever, just a few jangled nerves."

"Now the part I was debating about. It was my ward and I was on duty. It must have landed about ten to fifteen feet from me. I was at the desk and got up to get my jacket and helmet when I heard the incoming rounds. I always bring it with me when I come on night duty. The desk is about seven feet from the door, which is where the thing hit. Fortunately my path took me away from the impact just before it hit. I wasn't in danger. I do think somebody up there likes me. Anyway, now that it's over, it's just improbable that I will ever be that close again. I know that none of this will convince you that I'm okay and the situation here is really not that bad and only occasionally dangerous. I thought that you would want to know. If I had gotten a little scratch, I could have gotten a purple heart. That is one ribbon I never want to have. I never want to be that close again. It took about two hours for the butterflies to develop in my stomach. Before that I was just running around tending to business and escorting all the people that came over to investigate the situation. I reckon we're really in a war zone."

My mother is an extremely emotional person and she had a heart problem. I promised her I would be honest. Before I went I told her that I was probably safer in Vietnam in a war zone then I had been on the

Pennsylvania Turnpike. I had been on recruiting duty in Western Pennsylvania for two and a half years and frequently had to be on the turnpike.

I had requested to go to Vietnam but I never told her I had. I waited until my orders came in and then I called her and said, "Guess what? I got orders to Vietnam. I'm so excited." Take care and try not to worry. Lightening never strikes twice I'm told. I'm not worried. Besides that somebody said to me, "You must have gone to church on Sunday." I really do believe that somebody up there likes me and looks out for me. With that type of care why should I worry?

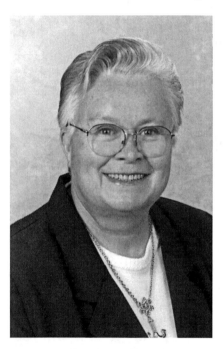

Lou Ellen Bell, 2012.

31 March 1969—"Life goes on as usual here in Vietnam. The hospital hasn't been that busy so we're going back on eight-hour shifts (from 12 hour shifts) as of tomorrow. Hope that it isn't an April Fool's joke. It could be that if we suddenly started getting a lot of patients we will have to go on longer shifts again. Let's hope our men don't get into that kind of action, for their sakes, not ours. We never put in the kind of work some of these men do.

As I walked to work this morning, I was listening to the singing of the birds. Apparently it is spring here. We haven't heard any birds until recently. Anyway, walking along in the quietness of the early morning and listening to those birds it's hard to remember that this is a war zone. I am only reminded when I see the injured or hear the bombing. Not much longer before I leave this job for someone else. By the time you receive this letter I will have begun my last one hundred days. If all goes well, it should go rather fast."

29 April 1969—"Just a note to let you know that I'm fine. Charlie welcomed our boss (Captain Bulshefsky, director of the United States Navy Nurse Corps) with a couple of attacks in the neighborhood community, so we went on alert. I'm certain she didn't get much rest. All was quiet for a couple of days and then tonight we had two more alerts. They were throw-

ing stuff at MAG16. I don't know what was getting fired on the second time, but all we received, in the way of patients, were Vietnamese. On the first alert we got several sergeants that were watching the outdoor movie at their club. I was having dinner with a friend over at MAG–16. We had steaks almost ready when the incoming rounds started. Needless to say I went into a bunker and he went to work."

28 April 1969—"I had lots of news to tell you but because of some of it I don't know when this letter will reach you. The ammunition storage area near Da Nang Airbase exploded yesterday as the result of a brush fire. Anyway, the resulting multiple explosions closed the air base to all fixed-wing aircraft. Some helicopters were landing, however. Some of these blasts were so strong that the buildings were falling from quite a distance around them because of the shocks from the blast. These buildings in some areas are not that sturdy. One of the hangars collapsed. The Freedom Hill exchange reportedly flattened. The First Marine Air Wing area had to be evacuated. You know from your map we are some distance from the air base. We only heard the blast and saw the smoke."

"I understand we did receive a massive number of patients as they had to be evacuated from the first hospital located there. We also got some of their doctors and corpsmen." They had no female nurses there. This was a first line hospital. It was a Navy/Marine Corps facility but it was staffed by doctors and corpsmen only, unless they had a male nurse anesthetist, which they might have. "We also got some of their doctors and corpsmen hopefully to augment our staff. Again there were no injuries as result of explosions. Well, I think this brings me up to present. The immediate future should be interesting. I am going on the hospital ship *Repose* for a couple of weeks starting Tuesday."

7 May 1969—"I am sitting in a cabin on the top bunk on the USS *Repose*. I came aboard yesterday and will only stay through Saturday or Sunday. I came out by helicopter, but I don't know about my trip back. I am working on the neurosurgical and the plastic surgery ward plus another ward that has all medical patients. I really like the ship. It would not have been bad to be stationed on board. But, there are some advantages to being stationed in Da Nang."

After 7 May 1969—"The puppies sound so cute (my dog had died and they had bought a couple of others). It won't be long before I see them. The flight dates haven't been published yet, but there is a possibility that I may be leaving a few days before the 15th. I have been packing so I could

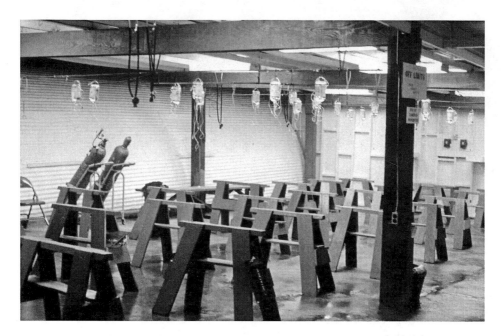

An admitting or ER department.

send my gear next week. I have been anxious to leave. I am a little reluctant to go now. I have worked with these kids (nurses and other staff) for a year and it is difficult to split up."

I left Vietnam in July 1969. I left a little early. I was scheduled to leave the July 15 and I got out a little bit earlier than I planned. I didn't quite get to the end of my 100-day calendar. We had to leave within five days of arrival of our replacement and mine got in a little early. We couldn't wait. We had to go. At that point, because I wasn't going to school until August, I had all of June and July before I went to school. We were pretty busy at the time I left. In fact they had sent some extra nurses to supplement the staff. So, I said to Helen Brooks, "Is there any possibility that you could request that I stay a little longer since I don't go to school until September?" She said she couldn't.

Lou Ellen came home and completed her Navy time to retirement. After retirement she worked many years as a civilian nurse in home care. She continues to be active in the Navy Nurse Corps Association.

Karen Born

Karen's account speaks to the difficulties of working in a wartime situation, but also developing positive relationships and good memories.

I began my Navy career in 1968 at San Diego Naval Hospital during the Vietnam era. I quickly understood part of my job was to provide the student corpsmen with opportunities to develop skills and confidence because most of them would rotate through Vietnam eventually. I enjoyed teaching and helping the men understand when they attached to a Marine Corps unit they would have a great deal of responsibility. Hospital Corps School was originally 16 weeks long but, as the war progressed, it was shortened to ten weeks. The students had two weeks on the ward during which they gained some hands-on experience. I was teaching all the time, "You must do your best because your life and the Marines' depend on you." Necessity required these young men to mature quickly.

My primary duty was on the neurosurgery ward. When we worked evenings, we had to run two wards, both neurosurgical. When we worked nights, we had three units, two neurosurgical wards and an ENT (ear, nose and throat) ward. That's when I learned about patients with their mouths wired shut due to different facial fractures. They ate liquid food meals through a straw. You'd be surprised what they would mix up so it had some taste. The men used to order pizzas which they pureed in a blender with a little tomato juice.

I was concerned when I learned I was assigned to the neurosurgical ward. I had not received any neurosurgery experience in college. My school felt it inappropriate for nursing students because it was so exacting. I thought, "Oh good, here I am working with corpsmen on a 48-bed open ward and I have never taken care of any of these kinds of patients before." I quickly became educated about Striker frames and circle electric beds, how to turn the patients and keep them safe, and all the varying injuries with which the patients were returning from Vietnam. My corpsmen taught

43

me so much. At that time the military still had the draft so we had a lot of well-educated high school and college graduates suddenly in the Navy as corpsmen. They were really nice guys and very willing to teach me the techniques needed to provide appropriate patient care.

My orders said I was supposed to be in Vietnam on January 15. I went from home in Ohio back to the West Coast and caught my scheduled flight. We stopped on Wake Island and Guam on our way to Vietnam. As we were landing in Da Nang, the pilot announced it might be a little bumpy. An hour earlier there had been a mortar attack on the runway and they hadn't had time to fix the mortar holes yet. I thought, "Oh shoot, the runway got fired on. This really is a war zone but I'm going to a ship; I'm not really in a war." We got off the plane and I looked around for someone who was supposed to pick me up. I had been assured I would be met and taken to the location where I would catch the mail boat out to the hospital ship, USS *Sanctuary*, AH–17, which would be in Da Nang harbor. There wasn't anybody there. I started talking to other people who suggested that maybe my greeter was waiting for me at the pier. The veterinary technicians had their trucks at the airport because they were picking up some dogs so they offered to drop me off. At the boat pier there were a lot of military members who had come ashore and were waiting to go back out to their ships. We could use our one day off each week to come ashore and go to China Beach, the officer's club or other places. Someone finally pointed out the *Sanctuary*. I was picked up and headed for the ship.

The water was rough and salt water was splashing all over us. By the time we reached the ship, I and my luggage were soaked. Ladies were supposed to go off first. Obviously when you're wearing your summer blues, you've got on a skirt. We had no pant suits at that time. The guys wanted you to go first so they could kind of "peak" under your skirt. The officer of the deck took me down to the chief nurse's office where the chief nurse said, "You're a day late." I said, "No ma'am, I don't think so. My orders said I was to leave on the 13th. I left on the flight I was assigned." She had totally forgotten about the International Date Line. She expected me on a certain day and I arrived a day later. That is why she had nobody to greet me. She was already reporting me for "missing movement."

I got aboard the *Sanctuary* around 1600. Junior officer meal time was at 1700, so I had an hour to get my "stuff together." I reached my room and found so much salt had gotten into the locks of my luggage I couldn't get the suitcases open to get out dry clothes. One of the other girls said to me, "Take your uniform off quickly and I'll throw it in the washer and dryer." Somebody else took my suitcases and was trying to get one of the engineers to see if they could get the salt out of the locks and get them open. I wore a very warm, wrinkled but dry uniform when I went to eat. I had my dinner in the officers' mess and then came back to the nurses' quarters to meet my roommate and others. I learned I was assigned to neurosurgery because of my experience.

I had a wonderful time in Vietnam. We worked hard and played hard. The patients reminded me I was in a war zone but I only remember the good times and dedicated shipmates. I worked neurosurgery for a while. Just like stateside, if you worked the day shift, you worked only one ward. If you worked PMs, you worked neurosurgery, urology, ENT, and the Vietnamese ward where we had women and children. When you worked nights, you had two complete decks. I could be responsible for a couple of hundred patients. There were one or two corpsmen working each ward and the nurse went from ward to ward as quickly as possible. The protocol said a nurse was the only one who could hang an antibiotic and almost all of the patients were on antibiotics. Each ward gave their antibiotics at slightly different times so you could get from one to the next. I'd hang the antibiotics, count the narcotics, administer pain meds to patients who needed them and run to the next ward. If you were working one of the days we were in Da Nang Harbor and had any patients being medevac'd, you had to make sure the charts were organized, signed off and ready to go by 0600. It was a very busy night for one nurse. It's a wonder we survived it, but we did.

After a while I was moved to the medical unit and SOQ (Sick Officer's Quarters). The medical unit had patients stacked three high in bunk beds. There were 80 patients on the medical ward and 20 on SOQ. The medical ward patients had malaria, dysentery, foot rot and cardiac problems. It seemed very strange to me to have cardiac patients in the midst of all this.

On medicine and SOQ I was working with my new roommate. We made it a lot of fun. An example of this was that on the end of every bunk was a little container with a life jacket in it. Because we had to take temperatures on all the malaria patients every four hours we would take the whistle out of the life jacket, blow and go, "Hey, everybody, listen up. Take out your thermometer, shake it down, put it in your mouth and the corpsmen will come around to check it." The thermometers were at every bedside taped in a plastic syringe container filled with alcohol. We still used glass thermometers then. We taught each patient how to shake it down and place it in their mouth. The corpsmen would walk by, record the temperature, check their pulse, replace the thermometer back in the plastic container and move on to the next guy. The chief nurse thought this was very unprofessional. She felt the nurse should go to each bedside, call the young man by his name, take a look at him and talk to him. When you had up to 80 temperatures to take, orders to transcribe, and other things to do, going to every bedside and talking to each patient every four hours was a little difficult. We used the whistle for quite some time until she told us we couldn't do it anymore. So we kept a lookout and blew it unless she was coming. I think most of the staff did this. I learned it from somebody who had already been there. It was one of those tricks we passed along.

SOQ is where I was introduced to the term "fragged." We had an officer that came in with shrapnel in his backside. I asked, "How did that happen?" Someone informed me his men wanted to get rid of him so they fragged his bunk. They put a grenade under his bunk and let it go off. I think I saw two cases of fragging during my year tour which convinced me it was a true story. The patient denied that's how it happened but, when I asked privately, he admitted it. I don't know if he understood why but he probably could have told me who he thought responsible though he never did.

I was also introduced to "friendly" fire shooting of corpsmen when a corpsman arrived on board with his hand damaged. Somebody in his unit thought he wasn't doing a good enough job so wanted to make sure he had an injury that would keep him from being out in the field. I think it blew off a finger. As I was talking to him I was reading between the lines. The patients won't tell you unless you figure it out. He expressed relief about being returned to the States. Some of the guys were so scared. Not everybody is macho. A lot of men chose to be corpsmen because of their "conscientious objector" status. Then they found themselves in the middle of a foreign country being shot at anyway.

The majority of the patients recovered from malaria or jungle rot and would be shipped to Cam Ranh Bay, which was an R&R (rest and recuperation) center. They got a couple more weeks rest before being sent back to the field. A lot of surgical patients got to go home while many of the medical patients just got well and went back to their units. I had mixed feelings about patching these guys up and making them feel better while knowing they were going back to the war. I could only hope they made it.

The sickest orthopedic patient was usually in the middle of a three-level bunk bed so he was the easiest to reach. As they got better they went to the bottom so the staff could still provide care. As the men were recovering they went to the top because they were a little out of sight and had to have some mobility to get up and down. I was having discipline trouble with one of the orthopedic patients who needed an antibiotic injection. He fussed with me and the corpsman. The doctor arrived for rounds, heard the noise, inquired about the situation and listened to our explanation. He took the syringe, went over to the patient and shot it right through the pajamas into his thigh. He emphatically instructed the patient to stop giving the staff trouble.

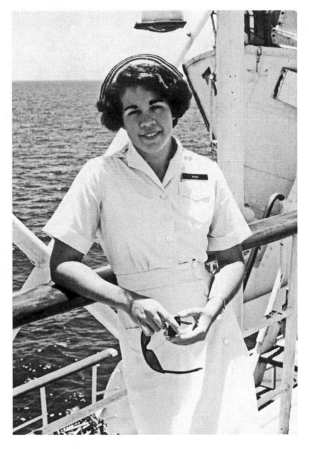

Lieutenant JG Karen Born aboard USS *Sanctuary* July 5, 1970.

On the Vietnamese ward, several children had a history of polio. One of our orthopedists was doing surgery to straighten their crippled limbs. Because the Vietnamese were used to squatting over a hole in the ground, when they saw toilets they would stand on the seat and squat over the bowl. We were constantly cleaning up because there was urine everywhere. The bathroom was the worst part of the job because it took some training for them to understand how to use a flush toilet, but they did figure it out.

There were several typhoons during my year on the ship and we always tried to steer away from them. I remember a stormy night I was working

47

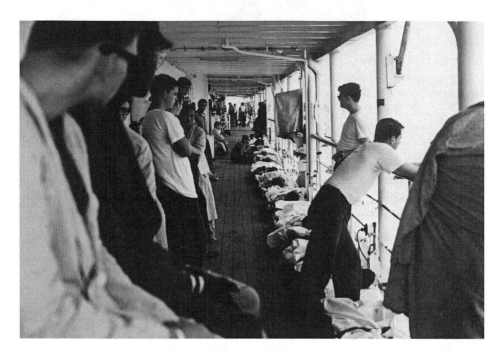

Patients lined up, awaiting medical evacuation from USS *Sanctuary*, July 1970.

and got really seasick. One of the corpsmen finally gave me a shot of Dramamine. For an hour the corpsmen didn't know where I was. They found me asleep on a bench as a consequence of the medication, woke me and got me back making rounds although I was way behind. It did cure my seasickness by working nights. I've always been a night person. I liked working nights except there were so many patients needing care.

I remember another rough, stormy night shift. Chest tubes back then consisted of a glass collection bottle on wheels. We would tie the unit to the bunk with gauze so it wouldn't roll around. I was making rounds and realized the gauze holding the collection unit was about to break. I hollered for the corpsman to come help me as I blocked the chest tube unit wheels with my foot while holding onto the bunk because the ship was rocking. I didn't want the chest tube yanked out of this poor kid. Just then the dressing cart broke loose from its ties and came rolling down the aisle between some of the bunks. It was about to crash into a bunk and all of the contents would land on the broken legs of another patient. I caught it with the other foot and one arm. I'm screaming for the corpsman, who is

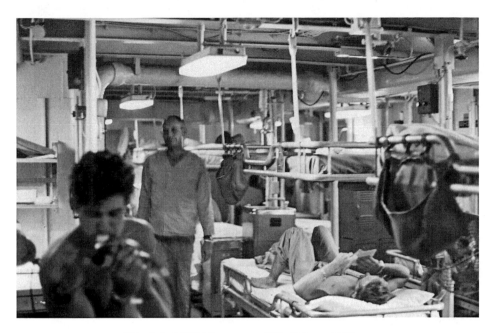

Ward A–3 USS Sanctuary AH–17 June 1970.

taking his good time getting there, and he wasn't far away. He finally arrived and helped get everything secured in place.

The ship's sailing pattern was three days in Da Nang Harbor, two days cruising off of Eagle Beach, which was part of Northern I Corps, and two days off of China Beach. We had to be cruising all the time to prevent someone from attaching explosives to the hull of the ship. When we were moored in Da Nang Harbor, they had river boats constantly patrolling the waters looking for divers. All night long we could watch the boats circling the ship.

We alternated schedules with the USS *Repose* which allowed us to accept wounded directly, so the Army field hospitals wouldn't get over-whelmed with casualties. During the day the hospitals would empty out those who could be flown by helicopter out to the ship, particularly the patients needing further treatment outside of the war zone. This would usually be about 30 to 40 patients. That way, during the night, when there were fire fights, the field hospitals would have empty beds to cope with fresh casualties.

Helicopter pilots preferred not to fly at night. Some Army helicopter

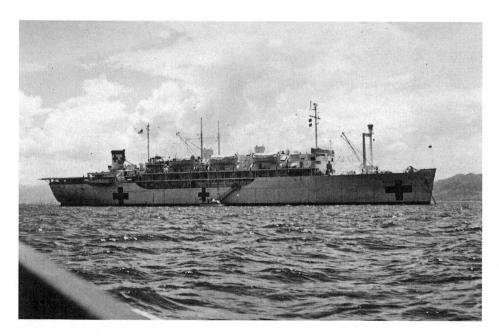

USS *Sanctuary* AH-17 August 21, 1970.

units would send a representative out to the ship, hang up an invitation, and the first five of our 28-nurse compliment signed up could go in-country to socialize with the men. At first I recognized it was the same group of girls going all the time and thought that wasn't fair. There was some kind of deal, one girl would hear about it and she would sign up her friends. At some point I got there first and listed myself and my roommate since I knew we would be off duty. On the scheduled evening, the helicopter flew out to the ship's helicopter pad and picked up the five women. We were in our summer blue uniform of a skirt and jacket with our legs showing. The reason the men invited the Navy nurses was because we had "legs" and the Army nurses didn't because they wore fatigues. I quickly learned to bring along a civilian dress. We had to leave the ship in uniform and arrive back in uniform but could wear civilian clothes if we were on a base in-country.

My first visit was with a nice group of pilots at Camp Eagle. We went to their "O" club and spent time with the helicopter pilots. We were just supposed to sit and chat with them, and if they had music, we could dance. They fed us supper. When we arrived at a unit, they'd take us to the CO's or XO's hooch (quarters) where we would change into our dresses. We were required to be back on board the ship by 2200 because the ship would move further out from the coast and steam all night to deter any swimmers from getting near. They started gathering us up about 2130 so we could change back into our uniforms while they started up the Huey helicopter. One nurse brought perfume so I put just a few drops under the CO's pillow. I thought the evening was very nice and wondered how I could send the men a thank-you note.

The next time there was an invite, it was to a different group at Camp Evans. I wrote a thank-you note ahead of time, applied some perfume to the note and took it with me. When we left, I put the thank-you note under the pillow. The CO contacted me and said, "Nobody has ever done that before." I said, "You guys were really nice to us." They fed us steaks for dinner. Every Sunday the enlisted men on the ship got steaks. The officers got steaks every second or third week. I thought it was interesting the in-country units got so many steaks.

These men got to know me because I was leaving thank-you notes every time. Then they started sending their representative out to the ship and instead of going to see the chief nurse, they would announce over the loudspeaker, "Would Lieutenant Born please report to the helo deck or the chief nurse's office.'" They would hand me the invitation and ask me to select five girls to come ashore. I was more selective than the original five who were going all the time. I set up some rules, such as, "You have to stay in the officer's club. You have to talk to any guy who wants to talk with you. You have to dance with anybody who asks you to dance. You have to be nice to everybody." There were many men in the unit so you couldn't pick just one. The guys seemed to like these rules. I said, "We're all in a war zone. Let's just act like ladies and not reflect poorly on the Navy Nurse Corps."

After we had been going to these parties for a while, we got to know the men in the groups. I would start asking about the guys that were missing since they didn't usually fly at night. I was told the men were in their hootch because they had to give up their steaks for us. They were hiding in their quarters eating K–rations. I said, "Now that's ridiculous. I'll share my steak. Bring the men back." When I'd see girls who would eat two or three bites of their steak and be done with it, I'd chastise them, remind them of the men's sacrifices for us, and let them know I didn't like their playing games. They were surprised I'd figured out men were missing.

Sometimes I wanted to contact these pilots. When I was on the ship, I needed to get a hold of them to say "Hi" or "Thank you" or "Are we still on for Sunday night or Friday night?" or whatever. We had a MARS Radio Station on the ship which only worked after 7:00 P.M. That's when it was the right time back in the States for families to answer their phones. You signed up to schedule when you wanted to call home. There was an E8 running the station at that time. Before starting calls to the States, he had to get on the radio at 6:00 P.M. with other in-country operators to share information or messages. You had to be careful what you said because you never gave dates, times, or locations, etc. I learned this and told him I wanted to be able to talk to some in-country friends. He said, "I'll make you a deal. I'll let you call them and I'll show you how to do it, but I eat dinner at 6:00 P.M. So, a lot of times I have to miss my evening meal or I get there late because I have to be on the radio. You take the in-country messages and then you have until 7:00 P.M. to talk to the pilots. At 7:00 P.M. I'll be back to start the MARs calls for everybody on the ship who wants to call home." On the days I wasn't working PMs, I would get on the radio. The first few times I was on, the reaction was, "Is that a skirt?" "Yes it is." "Where are you?" "Can't tell you. That's classified." I would record the messages and then speak to the COs and XOs of the different helicopter groups I'd gotten to know.

This was the beginning of Born's Helicopter Service. Crew members would be authorized to go on R&R but were often many miles out of Da Nang with no way of getting there to catch the R&R flight. Occasionally they would miss their R&R. Sometimes they would ask to remain in Da Nang for a day or two because they were supposed to catch a flight. Other times they would just try to figure it out or try to catch the flight which brought us mail. Shipmates started learning I was in contact with pilots, so they would ask if I could arrange flights for them. I'd dial/radio somebody up and ask if they could help with transportation. The crew wanted to know how I managed this. All you had to do was be nice to the pilots and sincerely thank them.

Eventually even the chief nurse came to me and asked for assistance in catching her R&R flight. She said, "I don't understand this. Just what do you girls do when you go ashore?" I replied we are there entertaining the guys by just being nice and sociable. We put on a dress, some jewelry and act feminine. Finally we took her in-country with us because she asked to go. It was very intriguing. I told the CO of the group we were bringing the chief nurse so he got a colonel to escort her. The colonel took her in his jeep for a tour of the camp and did a good job of entertaining her.

Then a storm came in and all of sudden word came flights were grounded. They couldn't get us back to the ship on time. We women ended up sleeping in the CO's quarters wherever we could find a spot. We radioed the ship to remind them five of us were in-country and wouldn't be able to return until the storm passed. Eventually the weather started to clear and we were awakened at two or three in the morning. They wanted to get us back to the ship since it was starting a course back to Da Nang. That meant the pilot had to fly us a lot further in bad weather to join the ship than they would have normally. We were all in a situation where we were going to miss movement. I wondered how much trouble could we be in. We've got the chief nurse with us. We did finally get back to the ship, finished sleeping through the night, and got up to do our duties in the morning. Nothing catastrophic had happened.

Most of my pictures of Vietnam are from the air because the pilots would include us on noncombat flights. I'd get to sit in the front seat of the gunship or the light observation helicopter and view the countryside. I'd see where the mortar rounds had hit and the domed Vietnamese burial sites, which were kind of above ground but under cement.

Every 90 days the ship would go into Subic Bay, Philippines, for maintenance, repair, and restocking. The trip took two days each way. We tried to medevac out and off-load most of our patients prior to leaving Vietnam. Some patients were taken to Subic for treatment or medical evacuation from there. Since we didn't have as much patient care to do, we did a lot of scrubbing and cleaning. The ship had two commanding officers, one for the ship and one for the hospital in the ship. When we were in Subic Bay, the hospital CO and I did a lot of dancing because I was one of the taller girls and he was over six foot. He was a talented, smooth dancer so we would enjoy the bands and singers at the Subic officers' club.

I wanted to make fudge, but we weren't allowed to have any cooking facilities because of safety. I got to know the ship's captain steward. He had a hot plate where he prepared the captain's meals. I asked, "If I bought the ingredients when we were in Subic, could I make fudge?" and he agreed. It turned out the ship's captain could smell it. He sent a message via the steward he would not complain as long as every time he smelled fudge he found fudge on his dinner tray. Afterward I made fudge and made sure he got some.

Each officer had a safe that was part of the desk unit built into their quarters. Most kept money, valuables, or jewelry locked up. A few officers brought alcohol on board even though they knew it was illegal. Every few months we had unannounced inspections of our living quarters. The nurses were called over the loudspeaker to return to our quarters and stand at attention outside the door of each room. My room was on the open end of a U-shaped hall by an exit door and outside hatch. As the inspectors entered one room, someone else would be taking alcohol out of their safe and passing it down the line of all these women outside their doors. It would end up in my hands since I was the last one in line. I was supposed to sneak out the hatch and throw it overboard. I rarely drink so I got frustrated doing this. I spoke up and told the nurses, "If you're stupid enough to bring the alcohol aboard, then take the penalty that comes with getting caught." I was in Vietnam from January 15, 1300, 1970, to January 15, 1500, 1971.

I then returned home to Ohio and spent some time with my parents who were very supportive. I spent a lot of Christmases overseas during my career so they would just hold Christmas until I came home in January. The tree would still be up with the packages under the tree and we would celebrate Christmas in January.

Karen went on to complete her career in the Navy and retire to San Diego, California. She continued to use all the skill she had learned in the Navy as she extended her nursing career into the civilian community.

Mary Breed

The next two accounts are very personal stories of nurses' experiences actually on the front in Vietnam. They help the reader understand the physical and emotional situations nurses found themselves in when serving in-country during the war in Vietnam. They speak of a desire for education, nursing experience and adventure. They speak of naïveté about the war and the developing reality of the situation to each of them. They speak of love of patients, colleagues and country.

When the Tet Offensive occurred in 1968, I was a junior at Swedish Hospital School of Nursing in Minneapolis, Minnesota. This was when the Vietnam conflict, "war," became personal. My friend from church was killed in Da Nang. During 1968, my brother was wounded.

Because of the increasing number of casualties, the need for nurses increased and recruiters from the Navy, Army and Air Force came to all of the nursing schools in Minneapolis. My friend and I decided to join the Army to be "where the action was." Remember, we were the Kennedy generation: "Ask not what your country can do for you, but what you can do for your country." I joined the Army both for personal and patriotic reasons.

Basic training at Fort Sam Houston introduced me to Army life. The lecture on triage made me realize I was not ready for Vietnam. I started out in basic training at Sam Houston where we learned to work triage. I attended a nursing school where there were no male nurses in those days. During the training at Sam Houston I learned to put foley catheters in men. We never learned to do that during my nurses' training. There were male orderlies to do that. At Fort Sam we saw sucking chest wounds and we had to learn what to do. In those days the doctor had to be present when we hung blood. We didn't have the same responsibilities compared to today's nurses. But that would be different in Vietnam. Although I graduated from an excellent school of nursing, I rarely saw trauma cases. In

Vietnam we would have some responsibilities only doctors had in the States. Vietnam would change the future of nursing.

After the lecture on triage, we were told half of our class would go directly to Vietnam. They said the Army was so desperate for OR nurses, they would offer us a three-month OR course tailored for Vietnam. This was an offer I could not refuse. I went to Fort Bliss in sunny El Paso, Texas.

The staff at William Beaumont General Hospital was wonderful. On the day of our final, our instructor called me to her office where she informed me everyone else received the assignments they requested. However, since I worked so well with civilian nurses, I would be going to Fort Jackson, South Carolina. The military's first priority for nurses was overseas and so many military hospitals in the states were staffed with civilian nurses. Fort Jackson needed one more military OR nurse. They already had one colonel and one captain. To say the least, I was very disappointed.

When I called my parents, I was crying. My dad told me I joined the Army for the right reasons. He suggested if I didn't like it I could put in my two years and get out. About an hour after he hung up I received phone call from a colonel at Fort Jackson. As the colonel welcomed me to the hospital, I recognized my Dad's voice. When I started to laugh, he knew I'd be okay. The irony is my Dad left for the Philippines from Fort Jackson during World War II. The five months at Fort Jackson flew by and after returning from a friend's wedding in California, I was told I was going to Vietnam. I couldn't believe it.

Following a short leave at home, on September 3, 1970, I was off to Travis Air Force Base where I boarded a civilian plane for my flight to Vietnam. I was so glad my friend, another Army nurse, had missed her first flight due to a luggage mix up. Besides the stewardesses, I believe we were the only two women on the flight. My friend asked me why I was hand carrying my OR book. I told her I had not done neurosurgery in the last five months and just in case I needed a review, it would come in handy.

Once we could see the coast of Vietnam, the whole plane became very quiet. Reality was sinking in. The air that hit my face as I stepped off the plane was unbelievably hot and musty. It was late at night when we finally arrived at our sleeping quarters in Bien Hoa. The building was surrounded by concertina wire and a guard was stationed at the entrance. I'm not sure if he was there to protect us from the enemy or our own men. My friend and I decided to share a room and leave the lights on since we were the only ones in this strange place. Upon waking from a deep sleep, my eyes opened to a ceiling full of bugs and lizards. I was horrified and took a quick walk outside. The guard said, "Ma'am, do you know what time it is?" He then informed me it was only 0200 and nothing was open at this time. I didn't want to make his night more miserable, so I went back inside.

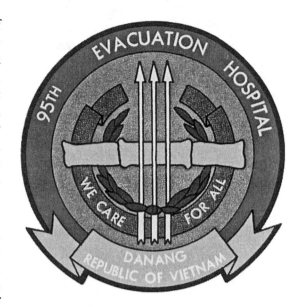

At 0600, after showering in a very filthy shower, we ate breakfast and went to see the chief nurse. I had been told I could choose the hospital I wanted and of course I wanted to be with my friend. Instead, the chief

Logo for the 95th Evacuation Hospital, Da Nang.

nurse said, "Lieutenant Breed, you're going to the 95th Evacuation Hospital in Da Nang. It is the neurologic center of I Corps." My friend knew I didn't want to do neurology and started laughing. The chief nurse looked at her and said, "Lieutenant, I don't know why you're laughing. You're going with her."

In Da Nang my hooch on the first floor wasn't kept up very well. When it rained, the water would leak into one side of the room where there were only slats and screening. Frogs loved my room. I heard some rooms had snakes so I tried not to complain. I had another wall that was not complete. Since I didn't drink or smoke, I used my PX card to buy liquor and cigarettes to barter for wood and other building materials. My corpsmen did the handy work and I enjoyed my new wall. Later, when I moved up to the second story, I decided I wanted to make my room more feminine so I used food coloring to make my walls pink and I ordered a pink flowered bedspread from the Sears catalog. I also ordered roller skates.

In 1970, the 95th was located at the base of Monkey Mountain and had approximately 320 beds. When I reported to the chief nurse, I was told I would spend time in admitting/ER before I started in the OR. I had to learn many new skills. Thank heaven the admitting staff was so patient and kind. At this time, we were working 12-hour shifts, six days a week and had one day off. Those who worked Tet in '68 did not have this luxury.

Some of my memories from admitting include treating Vietnamese children, adult villagers and occasionally missionaries from local orphanages. Treating children with white phosphorus burns, serious wounds, tetanus and other diseases brought joy mixed with much heartache. Once we had to evacuate the whole hospital due to a possible typhoon and I started to cry after the children were gone. A corpsman looked at me and said, "Lieutenant Breed, what are you doing? Nurses don't cry here." I said, "I do."

Admitting also included caring for GIs with malaria and other diseases. We triaged patients in the evacuation system and, of course, received fresh casualties. The wounded came from different countries including the United States, South Vietnam, North Vietnam, Australia and the Republic of Korea. Again the experienced corpsmen, nurses and doctors shared their knowledge with me.

My learning continued as I started in the OR. The first time someone said we were getting a "train wreck," I replied, "I haven't seen a train in Vietnam." Everyone in the room laughed. I found out a patient who was called a "train wreck" in Vietnam would have at least three or more services working on him at the same time. (Services include ENT, general, neuro, ortho, thoracic, and vascular.)

Two connecting Quonset huts made up the OR in Da Nang. There were six operating rooms. Each room only had three walls that provided some privacy. You could walk down the corridor and know what was happening in each room.

When there was downtime, we did cleft lip and palate repairs on Vietnamese children. It was rewarding to see these children smile. I worked with excellent, top notch people. Our OR team was made up of surgeons, CRNA's, corpsmen and nurses.

Because you worked 12-hour days, most nurses grew to love their corpsmen. Sometimes I would be the only nurse on duty and I knew my dependable corpsmen and respected their skills. Without asking, I knew which corpsmen would scrub neurology, orthopedics, etc. We became a family of sorts. It was an honor to be called "Mom Breed." I hope the families of my corpsmen know what a great job they did in such a difficult situation.

Besides the young casualties and deaths, what caused me added stress was the perception some men had of nurses. People that worked with me knew my values. They knew I believed in no sex outside of marriage. I would go out to the dinner with married friends, but that was all. I respected their wives at home. So, it really hurt me when one day a surgeon approached me at a party. He said he had an "open marriage." I asked who his wife was sleeping with that night. His hands came inches away from slapping my face. When I told him how insulted I was, he called me naïve. When I refused to go to bed with him a second time, he said I must be a lesbian. I told him I was not going to sleep with him to prove I was not. To say I was glad to see him return to the States is an understatement.

Another time, five casualties arrived in the OR. We were told it was a "frag a friend." A term I did not understand and thank heaven was not common. A group of GIs stopped in Da Nang on their way to R&R in Hawaii. Someone rolled a grenade into the room where they were sleeping. I was still new to 'Nam and used to make post-op rounds to see how our patients were doing. After three months in country, I did not routinely do post-op rounds because it was too sad. When I stopped in ICU, one of the nurses was trying to reach the R&R center in Hawaii to inform wives and others their loved ones had been injured. Then I went to the ward to check up on those less critical. It was there I heard what happened. It was terrible. They wanted to injure the lieutenant who ordered them to go back to an area where they had previously lost some friends. They were sad to hear a favorite sergeant died and were not sad to hear the lieutenant was critically wounded. Being upset, I said, "I don't know why I came here when we're killing our own men." One GI said, "You came here to get laid, like all the nurses."

With all of this going on, it's easy to forget the decent men who respected and protected me; my corpsmen, dust-off crews and, to my surprise, some men in the Air Force. One day, a few of my friends wanted to have Chinese food at the Air Force Base in Da Nang. After enjoying our dinner and conversation, we asked for the bill. We were told it was taken care of by the four gentlemen at another table. When we approached their table to say thank you, they stood up and said thank you to us for taking care of the wounded. There were no strings attached. It was exactly what I needed at that time.

In Da Nang I'd go to the officer's club to listen to music and occasionally dance to "Proud Mary" or We've Got to Get Out of This Place." I did sneak into the NCO club a few times. In Quang Tri there was only one club, which was good. After a bad or good day, everyone who wanted to, could go there. There were talented people who would play guitars and sometimes we'd sing along.

My drugs of choice in 'Nam were M&Ms and Coca Cola. Sometimes, I'd find my favorite drink, Grape Nehi, a kind of soda pop. I roller skated, played volleyball and board games, and read books. However, I never saw a complete movie. I went to the beach to swim, but could never learn to surf. My beach activities stopped after I saw water snakes. Sometimes on my day off, I'd hop a ride to visit a little orphan at the China Beach Orphanage.

Twice I made it out to the Navy Hospital Ship, USS *Sanctuary*. On my first visit, the Navy nurses gave us Army nurses a tour of the ship. I was surprised to see hammock-like beds stacked one above another. The well trained Navy corpsmen impressed me. After our tour we were invited to stay for lunch. I couldn't eat much because of the ship's movement. Some of the Navy nurses laughed because they said the ship was in port and it was not even moving. I grew to respect the Navy nurses as I listened to how strict the rules were and how confining it was on the ship. As I returned to land, I appreciated the people I worked with even more. I realized it was a wise decision not to join the Navy.

Many nights I would fall asleep listening to my reel-to-reel tape recorder. I enjoyed songs by Peter, Paul and Mary; James Taylor; Neil Diamond and songs on a special tape given to me by my corpsmen.

I took the war very personally as I saw how the terrible injuries would have a lifelong impact on the GIs, their parents, wives and children. When off duty, I remember just sitting, talking and crying with other nurses. When in my mind, things seemed really bad, I would remind myself I had it better than those who experienced the Holocaust. Since comfort came from my faith, I attended a few chapel services. Usually though I had my devotions and prayed privately inside my hooch.

The 18th Surgical Hospital had quite a history in Vietnam. By August 1968, when the hospital returned to Quang Tri, female nurses were reassigned. There was also a 40-bed children's hospital that was previously located at Dong Ha (Company D. 3rd Marine Battalion). The thing I loved about the 18th Surgical Hospital was it was a small unit. There were only nine female nurses.

Some of my memories from Quang Tri include the day choppers

landed both sides of the hospital and we received 75 wounded in 15 minutes, young men who could not see, hear, speak or breathe. Everyone worked hard, the cooks provided nourishment, and it seemed to me the grave crew quietly went about their duties.

One day I flew down to Da Nang to see a child in the orphanage. On the way back, I missed my flight at Phu Bai. Due to troop movement, all other air traffic was stopped. So, a nice young man from the control tower got his mattress so I could sleep on the side of

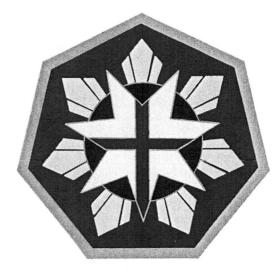

Logo for the 18th Surgical Hospital, Quang Tri.

the tarmac. He had offered me his hooch, but I was uncomfortable with that arrangement.

In the morning, I called Quang Tri to have a friend cover for me until I could make it back. She said there were no casualties at that time. I don't know how it happened but I heard a click and Colonel Johnson said, "Lieutenant Breed, do you know there is a war going on?" By the tone of her voice, I knew I was in serious trouble. I took the first jeep I could. Even though I was smelly and had bad breath, I took a ride with some Marines. As we drove through Hue, a beautiful city, I said I wished I had my camera. I'm not sure what camp they stopped at. All I know is when they dropped me off at the gate, I took the next available jeep.

The driver was an ROK Marine (Republic of Korea) who said he was going to Quang Tri. Suddenly he stopped the jeep and reached into the glove compartment. (Is he going to rape me? How much was I worth as a POW? I was bigger than he was. Could I outrun him? What about land mines?) When I saw him pull out some candy, I started to laugh. I thought of what my mother always said, "Do not go with strangers that offer you candy." He became highly offended at my nervous laughter and told me to get out of the jeep. As he drove off, leaving me in the middle of rice paddies, I was really scared for the first time in 'Nam.

Then I heard the sound of trucks coming in my direction and I didn't know what to do. Although I feared land mines, I stepped down into the rice paddy. Nothing happened. The first truck that passed me was full of Vietnamese soldiers. The second truck skidded to a stop shortly after it passed me and one of the two American GIs in the truck yelled, "Ma'am, do you know where you are? Where are you going?" I told them I wanted to go to the 18th Surgical in Quang Tri. As I hopped into the back of the truck, I could still hear swearing followed by "Ma'am" as they drove off. I wish I knew their names so I could thank them—to me they were angels! Colonel Johnson didn't reprimand me because shortly after I returned we received casualties.

One day a wounded pilot landed on our helipad. I don't know how he made it as he had a large blood loss and was having seizures. I hung blood for his case. On the way back to my hooch, I stopped at the chapel to pray. Because I didn't want another young man to go home and not recognize his family, I pleaded with God to let him die that night. The next morning Dr. Neuman, who knew I was upset by this case, had the pilot do math problems to prove there was no brain damage. To me, it was like God said, "Mary, you never decide who lives or dies in this war. You are here to do the best you can and that's all."

If anything good comes out of war, it's the increase in medical knowledge. Knowledge of septic shock, ARDS (acute respiratory distress syndrome/Da Nang lung) and PTSD (post-traumatic stress disorder) are a few from 'Nam. However, healthy young men die, in body and spirit. Vietnam showed me how a diverse group of people could work closely together as a team.

One day, as I was roller skating back into the compound, Colonel Johnson sent a jeep to bring me to her office. I figured she was displeased with me since I was being escorted. To my surprise, she appeared to have been crying. Out of nowhere a man from the Red Cross informed me my Dad had died. He had no details and repeatedly asked if I wanted to go home. I thought it was a foolish question. Of course I wanted to go home.

In a daze, as I walked back to my hooch crying, I said goodbye to everyone I met. Friends helped me pack. I don't know how I slept that night, but I did. The next morning at the airport, Colonel Johnson gave me an envelope filled with money. She said the guys from graves start the collection. I was shocked because I did not know any of them by name.

The money was to be used for the plane trip home because I had to pay my own way from California to Minnesota. Whatever was left was to be given to my Mother. Of course, I started to cry. To this day, that act of kindness can bring tears to my eyes.

I left Da Nang on June 9, 1971, on emergency leave and made it home a few hours before my Dad's funeral. I received an honorable discharge from the Army on July 15, 1971.

With God's help, love of family and support of friends, life has been anything but dull since 'Nam. I've enjoyed traveling around the world, even returning to Vietnam with Veterans Vietnam Restoration Project. I've kept in touch with other veterans through the Vietnam Veterans Association. The Vietnam Women's Memorial Project brought together a group of nurses from Minnesota and Wisconsin. We've become a "sisterhood" and get together at least twice a year. At the 95th Evacuation Hospital Reunion in New Orleans, I saw three of my corpsmen. I have met their lovely wives and always look forward to their yearly Christmas letters. Through the 237th dustoff reunions, I've met old friends and met one of our patients.

I will never forget the caring people I met in 'Nam.

Linda Caldwell

I liked science and math when I was in high school. I never really had a burning desire to be a nurse although I had read all the Clara Barton and Florence Nightingale books when I was younger. When I graduated from high school in 1962, the options open to women were very limited. I tell my daughters that you either went into teaching, nursing or became a secretary. If you were very good looking and thin, you could *maybe* become a stewardess, as they called them in those days. I don't think my girlfriends in high school really thought about going into medicine or other male-dominated professions. I don't mean to say that nursing was a second choice or a lesser profession. I just felt it was a good fit for my interests in science and math.

While I'm not Catholic, I attended the University of San Francisco (USF), a Jesuit school with the Sisters of Mercy serving as administrators and primary instructors for the School of Nursing. At the time, the only women students enrolled in the university were in the school of nursing, although shortly after I started they opened up all divisions to women. It was the only college I applied to, so in retrospect, I was lucky to be admitted. I was living in Las Vegas at the time because my Dad was in the Air Force. He was in World War II and when he got out he stayed in the reserves and got recalled during the Korean conflict. We traveled all over; Texas, Tennessee, France, England and then Nevada. I liked the military life; the fact that we had friends all over the world I viewed as a positive factor. As a military "brat" you learn to make friends easily, which I did and still do.

When I first went to University of San Francisco, I didn't think about going into the military. But a recruiter came to our sophomore class. He talked about this United States Army Student Nurse Program, and how the Army would pay your schooling plus give you a monthly stipend. When you graduated, you owed the Army three years of service. I felt it was a great option to pay for school. Having grown up in the military, I felt I had a good idea what to expect. So, I signed up and have never regretted the decision. There were several of us in my class that did, three or four girls out of a class of about forty. Some went into the Navy, but I decided the Army was my best option.

My parents were very supportive and proud of my going into the military. In December of my senior year I got my commission as a second lieutenant. I got a bump up in my monthly stipend. I think it was $200 a month, which in those days was a fortune! The Army also paid tuition, fees and books. I graduated in May 1966, and I took my state boards in June. In those days, there was no such thing as a computer. We sat for two days in a hotel in San Francisco and took the exams. You could work as a graduate nurse until you received your results, so I worked the 3–11 shift on a surgical unit at St. Mary's hospital in San Francisco, which is where I did most of my clinical rotations during school.

In August, I got my results, and shortly thereafter, I received my orders to report to Fort Sam Houston in San Antonio, Texas. I had to fly from San Francisco to Los Angeles and then to San Antonio. My flight left LA late in the afternoon and by the time we got to San Antonio it was around eight P.M. They fed everybody on the plane. When they got to my row I asked the flight attendant, "Don't I get a meal?" She said, "Oh no, you're military. You don't get a meal." I arrived in San Antonio really furious. I never did hear the rationale for that decision. I think I went to bed hungry that night. It was my first experience with discrimination against the military, which was something I'd never seen or heard during the time I was an Air Force dependent. I was in San Antonio for six weeks of basic training at the Medical Field Service School, the Army equivalent of boot camp for medical professionals.

In San Antonio I had a blast. There were nurses from all over the country. We went to classes during the day, learning military protocols, how hospitals were run, how to wear the uniform, how to march, and even how to shoot a .45 pistol. All the various branches of Army medicine went there for basic training; Army medical corps, nurse corps, and medical service corps (MSCs). We worked hard during the day, trying to learn "the Army way," and we partied at night. I still keep in touch with one of the women I met there and we've gotten together a few times since our days at "Ft. Sam."

Walter Reed Army Medical Center in Washington, D.C., was my first choice for a duty station after basic training and I was happy when I received orders to go there. I'd never spent any time on the East Coast, so it was fun to see a different part of the U.S., especially to be in our nation's capitol. I was assigned to a female medical ward, which was somewhat disappointing as I thought I'd be taking care of soldiers, not dependents. But I learned a tremendous amount and I actually enjoyed it very much. It was my first real work as a nurse and it was there that I learned how to start IVs and other basic nursing skills that we hadn't been allowed to do in school. I had a patient who'd been admitted with vague symptoms and no real diagnosis. She'd been with us a few days and was on every four hour neurologic checks. When I checked on her, one of her pupils had been "blown," just like in a textbook. I called the doctor and she was rushed to x-ray. That was in the days before CAT scans or MRIs, of course. I don't remember what the doctors found, but I felt good about my contributions to her care.

After a few months I was restless and felt I needed more in terms of learning experiences. Everyone except the head nurse rotated shifts; days, evenings, nights, and of course, weekends. My supervisor, a major, was a neat gal. She transferred me to the male neurosurgery ward. I loved it and felt I was really in my element! It was very hard work, but very satisfying. The patients were wonderful and made it all worthwhile. They'd tell you stories about being in Vietnam and that's when I started thinking, "I really need to go to Vietnam and see what this is all about."

We would occasionally get VIP visitors since our ward was a high visibility unit with 98 percent of the patients being returning Vietnam veterans. The guys, especially the guys on the Stryker frames who were paraplegics and quadriplegics, were alert and oriented. They could talk and kibitz. Pearl Bailey came to see the guys one Sunday, as did Mrs. Westmorland, the general's wife. She was lovely; a very, very nice woman.

We had a good group of nurses and we also had civilian aids, a couple of really great guys who helped us turn the heavy Stryker frames. I remember two older African American gentlemen who worked the 3–11 shift. They definitely kept spirits high for both patients and nurses when they sang "It Takes Two, Baby," which was very popular in 1967. They were a good group of nurses, corpsmen and aides with a lot of camaraderie. I was put in charge as a backup to the head nurse because in those days there weren't a lot of nurses with degrees. While the Army didn't require a degree, I guess they equated more education with more responsibility. I was evening charge and sometimes worked weekends on the day shift as the charge nurse.

I talked to the patients and they would tell me their stories about Vietnam. Some of them were really tragic. Back then a regular tour of duty in Vietnam was a year. You knew when you went you were going to be there for 12 months and then you could come home. That went for any-body, whether you were out in the field as a soldier or in a hospital. One of my patients had gone out with some of his buddies the day before he was to return to the States. He dove off a bridge into the river below and broke his neck, instantly becoming a quadriplegic. It was heartbreaking. We had one kid, the average age of soldiers in Vietnam being 19, who was admitted to our ward as a low-level quad. We all worked hard on his rehab and eventually he walked out of the hospital, albeit on crutches and very slowly. It was just absolutely amazing and we all cried when he left. Obvi-ously, not all the stories from that time were as good as his.

In the summer of 1967, I received a letter from the Army Nurse Corps Headquarters, saying I had been nominated to be an Army Nurse Recruiter by my supervisor, which was very flattering. They set me up with an inter-view in downtown Washington and essentially told me all I needed was a year of foreign duty before I could become a recruiter. I told them I wanted to go to Vietnam.

My mother had a lot of trouble with my decision. She respected my decision, but she was afraid for my safety, a woman going off to a war zone. My dad never talked about it, so I don't know how he really felt. I just know that they were very proud of me. At one point in time, my dad and I were on active duty together. He was a major and I was a second lieu-tenant.

I left for Vietnam the day before Thanksgiving in November 1967 from Travis Air Force Base outside of San Francisco. We left at night on World Airways, a commercial contract plane doing business with the mil-itary. I think there were one or two others nurses on the flight, but mostly men. We had to make an emergency landing on an island of the coast of Japan to refuel. We flew to Japan, the Tokyo military airport, to refuel and then to Tan Son Nhut AFB near Saigon.

I remember coming into Saigon in the daytime. They had warned us that we would come in at a very steep angle because they didn't want to give the Viet Cong too much access to the airplane, as in being a target for them. We landed and it was hot and steamy and a lot of different smells. I remember being so thirsty. There must have been a USO that gave us Cokes in glass bottles, which tasted so good.

It was Thanksgiving Day when I arrived and we were all taken by bus to the processing center at Long Binh and had Thanksgiving. I spent a couple of days there. Until I finally got orders for the 67th Evacuation Hospital in Qui Nhon on the coast of the South China Sea, which was south of Da Nang and north of Nha Trang.

There were a couple of us going to Qui Nhon. We flew at night, presumably because it was safer to move us at night. We flew on a C–130 and arrived very early in the morning. We went to the mess hall and had breakfast. Then somebody took me over to the nurse's quarters, our "hooch." I fell into bed and slept for eight hours. I was exhausted. I got up and started unpacking. I had a cot and a metal locker for my clothes, plus a metal dresser. When I got there, my roommate turned out to be a nurse who graduated a year ahead of me from USF. Talk about a small world! I arrived toward the end of November and she went home two or three weeks later, so we weren't together very long.

It was an interesting year. You get to Vietnam and you think, "Oh my goodness, I've got to be here for a year." There were highs and lows. There were days when you just said, "I want to get out of here. I can't stand this place." It is very confining. You think about working in a stateside hospital in those days, in the 1960s. You went home and you had friends and you went out and could travel, weekends off and do fun things. In Vietnam, we worked and lived with our coworkers. There was no escaping it. The only time you could get away is when you went on leave or R&R. After a while you bonded with everybody and they became your family.

The first couple of weeks it was tough. It was very different. The Army was very ill-prepared to have women in a combat zone. For instance, there was no place to buy any feminine hygiene supplies. Your family had to send it to you, a real care package if there ever was one. The PX, post-exchange, where we could buy various items—such as candy, gum, electronics, jewelry, etc.—didn't carry anything related to females such as cosmetics. One time I was down in downtown Qui Nhon and at the outdoor market someone was selling Cutex nail polish and lipstick, along with Sunkist oranges. Go figure!

The Sears catalog became our friend. I was 23 years old when I went there, and like most young women, you want new clothes now and then. I remember culottes were a big thing in the mid–1960s. While I was there, pantyhose came into being. Somebody sent me a pair of pantyhose. I thought these were the best things since sliced bread. We wore fatigues and combat boots every day. They actually were very comfortable and light-weight, which was important since it was so hot and humid in Vietnam.

Everybody had a "mamasan" to do your laundry, shine your boots and to clean your hooches. They came six days a week and we paid the princely sum of ten dollars a month. Every now and then my Mom would send me used children's clothing that her church had collected. I'd give them to my mamasan for her kids.

We had no hot water in our nurses' quarters. We had hot water in the hospital and the mess hall, but not in the nurses' or doctors' quarters. Each room housed two nurses with a shower, sink and toilet located between the two rooms. I shudder when I think about getting up every morning, taking a cold shower, washing my hair in cold water and shaving my legs in cold water. The mamasans washed our clothes in cold water; so needless to say, our white things didn't look very white after a while. I thought I had a tan until I went to Hong Kong and took a bath. It came off in the bath water. To this day I can't get into a shower unless it's hot.

In the hospitals we had hot water for the GIs and for our use there. In fact, when the patients would come walking in, the walking wounded, as we'd call them, they would go into the showers and they would be in there forever. I used to send corpsmen in to check on them and make sure they didn't drown. That is the first hot shower they would have had since they were out in the field. The doctors used to come up in their scrubs, wave and say, "Hi Linda, I'm going in to take a shower, just in case anybody needs me." Of course they didn't have beepers in those days. It never occurred to us as nurses to say, "One night a week, we are going to close the showers down. Nobody's going in there except the nurses." It never even dawned on us. As active and innovative and creative as we were, it just never occurred to us. We just accepted it. We were like, "Okay, we just take a cold shower." Obviously, women's lib had not arrived at the 67th.

When I went to nursing school, the nuns taught you to stand when a doctor came into the nurse's station and to give them your chair. You followed them around and did what they asked, no matter what. Not to belittle them in any way, because they did fabulous things, but that was just the way it was in the mid-sixties. Things were different in Vietnam and while we certainly respected them and their position, it was more of a collegial relationship. We were in the war and the situation together and we learned from each other, while maintaining a healthy degree of mutual self-respect. They relied on us to be their eyes and ears, almost like, and in many cases better than, interns. One of the surgeons I particularly respected was a great teacher and he taught me how to suture small fragment wounds. Obviously, it helped him out a lot because he didn't have to do it and could concentrate on the bigger cases.

I was head nurse of a 72-bed surgical unit almost from the time I arrived at the 67th. I didn't know what part of the hospital I would be working in until I went to meet with the chief nurse the day after I arrived. She told me they had an opening on the surgical ward, which was a relief as I didn't want to spend a year on a medical ward treating malaria and dysentery. The medical wards were never as busy as the surgical ones and I figured busy is better.

The mission of an evacuation hospital was to prepare patients for evacuation out of country, either to Japan or the Philippines, but mostly to Japan. Because our hospital was located alongside the Qui Nhon airfield, we had easy access to aircraft and daily flights out of country. Patients were hospitalized for approximately five days, which was about what it took to get them stabilized and ready to go. We were constantly admitting patients and discharging them, like a revolving door.

There were two hospitals in Qui Nhon. There was ours, the 67th, and the 85th. The 85th was further away from the air field. Their specialty was ears, nose and throat. They had an ENT surgeon. We had the only neurosurgeon in the area, so anyone with a head or spinal-cord injury came to our hospital, including Viet Cong prisoner patients.

Prisoners were admitted to our ward regardless of their condition, whether they were badly injured or had minor frag wounds. We kept them at one end of the ward, with a 24-hour armed Military Police (MP) guard. For the most part, the GI patients who were ambulatory would occasionally come to the prisoners' bedsides and try to talk to them in pigeon Vietnamese and English and would offer them cigarettes. Those were the days when you could smoke anywhere. A lot of the nurses smoked too, including me. For the most part, the GIs befriended these prisoners but we quickly assessed which GI patients to keep away from the prisoners.

Our 72-bed ward was devoid of privacy. There were 36 beds on both sides of the ward, with the showers, latrines, and utility rooms in between. The only privacy we could rig was with portable screens which we put around the beds whenever necessary. I don't remember the exact number of nurses who worked for/with me but it wasn't enough that we could work three shifts. Consequently, we worked 12-hour days, six days a week. Everyone was terrific and we all worked so well as a team. On the rare occasion our census was down, it was nice to close down one side of the ward and just operate out of one 36-bed unit. It was then that I could give the nurses an extra day off, which you also had when you worked the 7 P.M. to 7 A.M. shift. When you came off of that rotation, generally a six-night stretch, you got a "sleep day" as well as a day off.

Whichever side was busiest, I would be in charge and then I would assign the most experienced nurse to the other side. The prisoner patients were always just on one side of the unit because we only had one guard to watch them. The sicker patients, the ones who needed more constant watching, were located closer to the nurse's desk. We also had an intensive care unit (ICU) downstairs from my ward and next to the operating rooms (ORs).

The 67th had been originally been built to use as a barracks for the Air Force. It was really a very sturdy structure made of concrete with steel reinforcements. Located right on the airfield, it made a great hospital because the dust off choppers could land 20 yards from the emergency room or R&E (receiving and emergency). The hospital was a two-story structure with wooden ramps to the upper floors so they could push litter and wheelchair up to the ward. We had no addressograph plates, which were standard in all stateside hospitals in those days. As in any hospital, all the charts had to have the patient's name, rank, serial number, and date of admission on every single piece of paper. Talk about paper work! We'd often get 20 admissions at once (called a "regurg") and we didn't have a ward clerk to handle the paperwork. The nurses had to do it, generally me so that other nurses could assess and help admit the patients. We had great corpsmen and some of them were 91C3s, the military equivalent of a licensed practical nurse (LPN). They could do a lot more than just a regular corpsman, including their own charts, thankfully.

I was a head nurse of this surgical unit for eight months until there was an opening in orthopedics. The head nurse had finished his tour of duty and I asked to transfer to orthopedics. I wanted to do something different with my remaining time in Vietnam, to learn new skills and while I knew squat about orthopedics, I was blessed to work with two terrific doctors, a great team of nurses, and a super physical therapist. In addition to our GI patients, we also had a fair number of civilian casualties, including some children

One day after I'd been in country about six months, the Special Forces

(AKA: Green Berets) brought us a pregnant Montagnard woman. That's a French word meaning "people from the mountains," who were a gentle group of people, for the most part, and had different physical features than the Vietnamese. The Special Forces really liked them because they were good fighters and they trained the "Yards" to help fight the Viet Cong. This woman was in labor for a long time and presumably the Special Forces soldiers couldn't deliver her. They brought her down to the hospital because they knew we had a board-certified obstetrician on our staff. He'd been drafted into the Army and needless to say, he didn't get a lot of OB-GYN practice at our hospital. We teased him that he could put this event on his resume: that he'd delivered a baby in Vietnam. After delivery, they put mom on my ward to recover. I don't know where, but someone found a doll bed for the baby and we put her next to mom, who was in one of our regular cots with the privacy screen around them. She didn't speak a word of English, nor did we speak her language. We just communicated by sign language, which worked. This pair was a big hit with both the staff and patients and many photos were taken of them. A few days later, members of her tribe came and took her and the baby to their village. I often wondered how the mom and baby did and what stories the mom told her friends about us.

We had one little girl who was probably about ten years old. She had terrible strabismus. She couldn't see very well and walked into the path of a train. She must have been deaf, too. She lost contralateral limbs—her right arm and her left leg. We had her with us for many months and she was the sweetest little girl, very patient and very kind. She did well and we eventually transferred her to the local Catholic hospital for further care.

We had a little boy about four years old with a chronic, draining ear infection that was just disgusting. The thing I remember most about him is that he wouldn't wear clothes. My Mom and her church group had sent us boxes of children's clothes but he refused to wear them. He ran around naked and we nicknamed him "Pig Pen," after the Peanuts character. One day I had to take him to the ENT doc at the 85th Evac Hospital for a consultation. We went by ambulance and I held him in my lap. They gave him some sort of antibiotics and we kept him for a while until his parents came for him. I wonder if he ever got over his aversion to clothes.

Our favorite child was an 18-month-old little girl who pulled an oil lantern on herself and was horribly burned. She was initially hospitalized at the Catholic hospital in Qui Nhon, but the staff couldn't do much for her so they brought her to us. She was admitted with such bad contractures that she couldn't move her arm. She had lost one of her legs above the knee. Somebody on our ward started calling her Cindy, because she was burned to a cinder, which was awful. But she was really very cute, despite the scars around her face, and she had a very sweet disposition. Her family came to visit every Sunday to play with her and to bring her Vietnamese food. Cindy quickly became very spoiled. One of the corpsmen found a grocery cart (who knew we had such things on Army bases in Vietnam), so we put a pillow in the cart and sat her inside this grocery cart. We would wheel her from bed to bed and the GIs would entertain and play with her. We had a baby crib that she slept in during the night. She was our baby and we taught her how to salute with her remaining arm. We'd say, "Salute Cindy," and she'd whip out a salute. The orthopedic docs were just wonderful with her. They periodically took her to surgery to recast her arm, which eventually helped decrease the contractures.

While all my patients were special to me, the one from my days on orthopedics who stands out was a young guy, 19 years old, named Jim Baczkowski. "Ski" was out in the field, involved in a fire fight and had a traumatic amputation of his right leg. It was a very high amputation, what's called a total hip disarticulation. It happened four months to the day he'd been married. When he was admitted to our ward, he was pretty sick with a high fever and frag wounds, really in pretty bad shape. So we put him right next to the nurse's station. He was a really engaging kind of guy, with a good personality. I had a rule that before the patients left us for evacuation to Japan, they had to write a letter home. He kept saying to me, "I can't do this. I can't write a letter." He was 19 and she was 18 when they got married and he shipped to Vietnam a week later. I had such empathy for her and for him, of course. I thought, "How is she going to cope with this?" I asked Jim if he wanted me to write a letter to his wife. He said yes. I remember it wasn't easy to write that letter. Polaroid cameras had just come into being around this time and the Swinger model was a popular item at the PX. Someone took a picture of me with one of the corpsmen, which we put in the envelope with our letters and sent to with the letter. Jim was evacuated to Japan in late August 1968. A few months later, he sent us a letter and a picture of himself on pontoon skis, taken on a beautiful mountain in Colorado. He'd gone from Japan to Fitzsimmons Army Medical Center in Denver, which was the Army's amputee center. It was so rewarding to finally see a patient who made it back home and seemed to be doing well.

One night in March 1990, I was watching *Unsolved Mysteries* with my husband. It was one of my favorite shows and I always enjoyed the reunion stories. At the end of the program, they showed previews for the next week's stories. The host, Robert Stack, said, "Next week we'll show the story of a young Vietnam veteran who for 23 years has been looking for the nurse who saved him both physically and emotionally. Her name is Linda Sharp." Since Sharp is my maiden name, I was absolutely floored but felt it was probably someone else. However, I found the 800 number and called the show. A producer came on the line and asked if I remembered a patient named Jim Baczkowski, which of course I did. I was the "missing person!" It turned out that was the first time they had ever solved a mystery without showing the program itself.

After that, my phone started ringing with family and friends calling to say, "I think they're looking for you." I had started my new job at Schering-Plough, a pharmaceutical company in New Jersey, six months before this happened. My coworkers and management were very supportive of me and this amazing story. For several years afterwards, I was asked to speak about my experiences in Vietnam by several nursing organizations and civic groups. In all the years since I'd been back from Vietnam, no one had ever asked me what it was like to be a nurse there. It was as if no one really cared about nurses in Vietnam or what we did there until this publicity focused on the role.

Jim and his family were living Grand Junction, Colorado, with their two children, so the network (NBC) flew me out there and we filmed the update. That was an interesting experience in itself as I'd never done anything like that before. It was wonderful to see Jim again.

Jim was physically challenged but he wasn't handicapped. He rode horses, played golf, and built cars. He was an amazing guy and over the years that I came to know him after *Unsolved Mysteries* aired, things mellowed out somewhat. I think he felt better about himself but he still had demons left over from Vietnam. Unfortunately, those demons got the best of him and he died in 1998. His son called to tell me and while it wasn't a shock, it was nevertheless very sad. When I traveled for my job, I often went to Colorado and took a day or two of vacation to visit them. Jim's wife and I still keep in touch via email and we're forever linked by that special experience we shared.

Before I came home from Vietnam, I extended my tour of duty by a month. I was due to come home the early part of November but if I'd done that, I would have been starting my next assignment right before Christmas and I wanted to spend it with my family. During my last month in Vietnam, I took a five-day leave and went to Bangkok. I'd taken my R&R in Hong Kong in June so it was good to get away again for some "retail therapy." I still wear the jewelry I bought there.

I left Vietnam December 7, 1968, on an Air Force C–141 flight from Cam Rahn Bay, bound for Travis AFB in California. I wanted to go to San Francisco and see my friends from college before going home to Las Vegas, but if you left Vietnam on a commercial flight from Saigon or Da Nang, you went into the Seattle/Tacoma (SEATAC) airport. I had to wait several days in Cam Rahn Bay to get a flight but finally I got the message that the flight was leaving the next morning at 0700 hrs. I wore my fatigues and boots because I knew it was going to be a military plane and not the cushy commercial flight that would have necessitated my Class A uniform. As I entered the aircraft with about six or seven GIs, we saw that the back of the plane was filled from floor to ceiling with caskets. Years later, I was watching an episode of the TV show, *China Beach*, and that same situation was repeated. It was definitely a case of art imitating life.

When we landed in Japan to refuel, I was asked if I'd give up my seat for a GI going home on emergency leave. I did that and spent the next eight hours in the terminal waiting for another flight, which turned out to be a commercial aircraft. Not only was I the only woman on a planeload of GIs in their nice khaki uniforms, I was wearing my fatigues and combat boots. As the plane touched down at Travis, everyone cheered and clapped. I called a friend to come and pick me up. There were no cell phones in those days, of course, so I couldn't call ahead. When I walked into the terminal, there was nobody there to meet us. Conversely, there wasn't anybody throwing tomatoes at us either, calling us "baby killers." It was very low key. You were expected to get back to things the way they were. There was no decompression, no debriefing.

As for the recruiting job, I received a letter from the Army Nurse Corps headquarters in October while I was still in Vietnam with an offer to be the recruiter in Los Angeles. That appealed to me as my family was in Las Vegas and I'd be able to see them occasionally. Shortly thereafter I got another letter saying that the Los Angeles recruiter had decided to extend her tour and I was offered either Fort Benjamin Harrison in Indianapolis or Fort Des Moines in Iowa. After thinking about it for a nanosecond, I decided to decline the offer and asked to be assigned to Letterman

Army Medical Center in San Francisco. Fortunately, I got what I asked for.

I worked in ICU at Letterman for a short time until someone saw that I had a neurosurgery background so I was made head nurse of male neurosurgery. In March 1969, we opened the new, beautiful multi-story hospital which has since been torn down. There was a beautiful view of the Golden Gate Bridge from the day room but unfortunately, most of the patients couldn't enjoy it as they weren't ambulatory.

I got out of the Army in August 1969, which seemed like a good idea at the time. In retrospect, I've often wished that I'd stayed in and made a career of the Army. But I was tired of the military and wanted to work in a civilian hospital and wear my nursing school cap and different uniforms. Subconsciously, I think I was also tired of caring for all the young men with horrific injuries and wanted to see some "happier" aspects of nursing.

I met my husband and got married in 1971. He was an Air Force captain when we met and he's also a Vietnam veteran. We've been married 40 years, have three beautiful daughters, a granddaughter, and another one on the way. I used my GI bill benefits to get my master's degree in nursing at Rutgers University in 1980 and have worked in some aspect of nursing since then.

As far as lingering effects from my days in Vietnam, I'm very lucky. For the most part, my experiences were positive and I always say I'd do it again in a heartbeat. But I didn't work in ICU or the ER and see the really tragic cases. Yes, I worked with soldiers who were badly injured, but for the most part we got them to a better place and they went on their way. I often wondered how they did once they got back to the States. My postwar experience with Jim reminded me that not all wounds were physical. Some of the nurses who worked in ICU suffered negative effects, my roommate being one of them. It was hard to turn off your feelings, especially when you worked a 12-hour shift, six days a week.

I had some tremendous experiences and learned a great deal about myself and nursing during my year in Vietnam. What did I learn? If anything, I think you learned to deal with a bad situation and make the best of it, be innovative and creative, think on your feet and assess situations quickly and efficiently. You learned to set priorities and organize. You learned to do without a lot of things. We didn't have all the stateside amenities like pill cups and whatever. We would use the ends of syringes. The syringes in those days were encased in plastic with a cap that you twisted off. We used those as pill cups. Little stuff like that. You learn to conserve. You didn't know when you were going to run out of stuff. You weren't extravagant with things. It was just an awesome time ... a different kind of war. I think you could apply what you learned there into other areas of medicine. Every nursing experience you have you build on.

Alene B. Duerk

Alene B. Duerk became the first woman admiral in the United States Navy and the first admiral director of the United States Navy Nurse Corps. Her professional career crossed three wars. Her clinical experience involved every type of military health-care facility and every position of responsibility available to a woman during her time of service. Her early nursing experiences give much detail about the development of the profession of nursing and were essential to her preparation for her eventual position of leadership during the Vietnam War.

After graduation from nursing school I worked labor and delivery at Toledo Hospital. I felt very fortunate because jobs were hard to come by in 1941 because of the depression. I worked there for about five months. December 7, 1941, was Pearl Harbor Day. As a result, four of us, school classmates, decided to join the Navy.

When the war started, interns, residents and nurses were going into the military. The shortage was really very pronounced on the civilian side. I also had some family concerns, but my family and I felt I should go. It was a patriotic thing, service to country. I just felt I could do a lot more good in the military.

At the time the Red Cross was doing all the recruiting. The military didn't have recruiters. At graduation, our director of nurses had advised all of us to join the American Red Cross and most of us did. They called us many times, wanting to know which service and when we could go on active duty.

Finally, in the fall of 1942, I made application directly to the director of the United States Navy Nurse Corps. I wanted to become a Navy nurse. I got my commission in January 1943. As soon as I was commissioned in the United States Navy Nurse Corps Reserve, I got my orders for Portsmouth, Virginia.

I arrived at Bethesda in the morning about seven o'clock. I had been on the train all night. I was 23 years old. I had my physical and it was all over with by two o'clock. I can still see the chief nurse at Bethesda saying, "If we get her a cab now, we could still get her on a train to Portsmouth this afternoon." I thought the war was going to be over if I didn't get there immediately.

They put me in a cab. I went down and boarded the train and started for Portsmouth, Virginia. It got dark and I was still on the train. The train stopped and everybody got up to get off. I asked, "Is this Portsmouth?" "No lady. This is Newport News and you have to get on a ferry to go to Portsmouth." So, I trundled off with my two suitcases. I followed the crowd made up of all kinds of people going to Portsmouth. I got on this ferry. I had no idea what a ferry was. I had never been on a ferry. We went down the river and finally we came to Norfolk, Virginia. The pier was at Norfolk. It wasn't a shipyard. It was just a pier. The shipyard was in Portsmouth.

We got off the ferry. I walked to a drug store. I had a number to call which was for the nurses' quarters at Portsmouth. It was for a girl who had been my classmate in Toledo, Ohio. I told her I was in Norfolk and asked how to get to Portsmouth. She told me walk another two miles and get on the ferry, another ferry. I was still carrying my suitcases. So, I walked down there and got on the ferry. It was a nickel ferry at the time. We went across to Portsmouth.

We pulled into the ferry landing and I got into this huge cab. I said, "I want to go to the Naval hospital." He takes me to the old Naval hospital with the big steps and the pillars. I drag my suitcases up there and the officer of the day was there. I said, "I'm reporting in for duty." "At this hour?" It was about ten o'clock at night. He called the night nurse who took me over to the barracks. We lived in barracks and there were 20 people in this big open room with all these beds lined up. We had a bed, bedside locker, half a dresser drawer we shared with someone else, and half a pasteboard closet to hang our clothes in. You could not have anything on your bedside stand. You couldn't have any pictures. Every day you had to tuck everything away so there was nothing showing.

I hadn't had anything to eat so my friend took me to the kitchen in the dining room in the nurses' quarters. She got me something to eat and then she took me back to my room in the barracks. She and the others in the barracks gave me a Navy Nurse Corps cap. They put it on my head and said, "Now, you are a Navy nurse."

I went to work the next morning in my civilian uniform with my Navy cap. Sometime during that next two weeks I was measured and fitted for ward uniforms. At that time we wore the long stiff uniforms with the long sleeves and the wide belt and I had a cape. I was very tall, so my cape just billowed out there. There was a civilian lady in Virginia who made these uniforms. She would get the material, a twill, at small stores. She would have bolts and bolts of this. She would lay it all out and she would make sixteen uniforms at a time. Within two weeks I had the Navy uniforms.

The first morning I reported to the chief nurse who assigned me to a ward. The nurse I worked with on the ward was maybe two or three weeks my senior. She had her own ward. It was a ward where they had upper respiratory infections, called "Cat Fever." I had come from a civilian hospital where if the patient had pneumonia, they were isolated. If they had to have oxygen tents, they were put in a special room. We were with at least 60 patients in a huge, big old room. There was a fireplace at one end of the room. This was a Civil War hospital. The patients were on either side of the room and there was a row down the middle. They had oxygen tents and those people who needed close attention were brought closer to the nurse's station. The morning I got there was "field day." The beds were all moved to one side of the room and the corpsmen scrubbed the floor. Then, all the beds were moved back to the other side of the room. It was my first inspection. All I remember were those beds going back and forth.

I didn't know one patient from another, but I charted whether they had eaten their meals and vital signs. I think I was taking blood pressures by this time, a task which had originally belonged only to physicians. They brought in the food cart at noon. It had wells with food. One was potatoes and one was vegetables and one was soup. They had a tray with meat. Everybody came with their trays and filed along, and we stood back behind the cart and served the food. For the patients who couldn't, the hospital corpsmen or the nurses would dish up for those patients and see that they got their food. After they had eaten, trays were rinsed on the ward. Some of our wards had their own machine dishwashers and you had to wash your own dishes. The machines were very commercial. They had these big trays, wooden boxes, and all these trays were set in there and they would go through this steam.

It was assumed you knew how to take care of patients. I did. It was hands-on care; giving baths, feeding the patient, giving medications, changing dressings and doing procedures were just natural. They were things I had learned in nursing school. The most important thing, as far as the Navy was concerned, was that I learn how to fill out all the right forms. That hasn't changed. I was a quick learner. Within a few weeks I had my own ward and I was orienting the next nurse. It was a med-surg ward.

The ward staffing had one senior nurse and two or three junior nurses. The hospital corpsmen saw to it that patients got their showers and baths. At that time, patients had to stay at the hospital until fit for duty or medically retired. We had patients who were around for a long time. So, you put them to work. They had to sweep, dust, help with the food and help with the dishes. You were supposed to have somebody who was senior act as master-at-arms. In the civilian world you didn't have that. I had never worked with corpsmen. As far as supervising the corpsmen, I didn't realize how much they knew or how much education they had, but they seemed to be able to do anything.

We didn't have anything like antibiotics. The first time I saw penicillin, we gave it to a patient IV and he got 5000 units. We sat there and counted the drops. It had to go very slowly because we really didn't know what was going to happen. Of course, the patients reacted beautifully. They were well patients to begin with and then they had hernias or appendectomies or whatever. They just blossomed. They had no reason to be resistant or have an allergy. It was just a miracle drug, as far as we were concerned. We had sulfa before we had penicillin. We had sulfa when I was still in training. The first antibiotic we had was neoprontisil. That was a red pill. It caused the emesis to be blood red. Then, we had sulfa and people couldn't believe how fast the patients would react to those. They used the sulfa drugs in powders for things like wounds out on the battlefield when they got injured. We gave the sulfa drugs by mouth. We gave the penicillin IM and some IV.

In January 1944, I was transferred to Bethesda. I was at Bethesda until April 1945. By that time, I had signed up to go on a hospital ship. The bulletin went up and I signed it. The USS *Solace* was one of the old ones. I was on the USS *Benevolence*. There was the USS *Repose*, *Refuge*, *Sanctuary*, and *Bountiful*. They were commissioned in March and April of 1945. They were built in New York at the Brooklyn Shipyard. They had been liberty ships, as far as the hulls went, but they had been rebuilt as hospital ships. The *Solace*, however, had been a passenger ship at one time. Down in the lower level the bunks were in four tiers. The ward I was on had racks for two patients.

I went aboard in April 1945. While we were on board, we had VE (Victory in Europe) Day in May. We left Brooklyn and came down to Norfolk, through the Panama Canal and over to Hawaii. We were enroute to Japan. We didn't know it then, but we were being sent out there for the invasion of Japan. The invasion was supposed to come in October. We went as far as Hawaii, then Enewetak in the Marshall Islands. While we were in route from Enewetak to Tokyo in August 1945, the bombs were dropped in Hiroshima and Nagasaki. Our mission was changed and we went into Tokyo Bay and liberated the POWs. We didn't understand about radiation and fallout, but I don't think I was exposed to it. At least I have never had any side effects. I was in the Marshalls and out at sea when the bombs were dropped. They had dropped bombs before, so it didn't really mean anything, as far as I was concerned. I didn't really understand what an atomic bomb was or the devastation that it was going to cause.

We got into Yokosuka late in the afternoon of the day we arrived. A chief met me on P.M. duty and said, "We are going to take on prisoners of war." These were our people who had been prisoners of the Japanese, but when I talk about "ours" I mean Australians, British, Americans, Russians, all these different groups who had been in prisoner of war camps. Some of them were from the United States Army who had been on the Death March of Bataan and had been prisoners of war for four years. They had been moved from the Philippines to Japan. I was concerned about them coming because I didn't know if we were taking on 15 or 15,000.

There were two prisoner of war camps and they were right outside Tokyo, Shinagawa and Omori. They had already been partially liberated because planes had dropped clothing and chocolate. This was the last of August. The bombs had been dropped early in August.

We took on 1,500 patients that night and the next day. The hospital ship had 750 beds. The prisoners of war came in, were examined, given new clothes and dusted for fleas and other kinds of vermin. They were transferred to other ships for the trip back to the United States. A few were flown out. Within 36 hours we had processed this large number of patients and we had a full load and the POW camp was empty. Those people who couldn't be moved, who needed to be stabilized or fed, became patients. A lot of patients had berieri and had been starved and there was concern about tuberculosis. Our galley worked 24 hours a day.

We docked at Yokosuka and we kept our patients for about a week. Another hospital ship came along and took these patients aboard and took them back to the States. There were three hospital ships there. There was a Dutch hospital ship called the *Titulinka*, a United States Army Hospital ship called the *Marigold*, and the *Benevolence*.

Within a week and a half we needed to take on other patients besides the POWs. We took on patients from the fleet. We became "the hospital." There were no hospital facilities on land so we became the hospital. We were there until around Thanksgiving time.

Alene went on to serve at Great Lakes Naval Medical Center beginning in January 1946. She got off active duty and went on inactive status, going back to school at the Case Western Reserve Francis Payne Bolton School of Nursing for her bachelor's degree. She graduated with a bachelor of science in Ward Management and Teaching Medical-Surgical Nursing in 1948. In 1948, she rejoined the Navy Reserve when she realized she missed the camaraderie of the staff and patients. She was recalled in March 1951 when the Korean War began, serving again at Naval Hospital, Portsmouth, Virginia.

Alene worked on a ward for head injury patients for three months and was then asked if she would like to teach in corps school, which was on the Portsmouth Naval Hospital compound. She continued there for five years throughout the Korean War.

"B" school was for first class and chiefs, those who were going to independent duty. They were taught advanced procedures. I can remember teaching the nasal tube, the Wangensteen suction machine, sterile technique and different procedures that they might have to do aboard ship until they could get a patient stabilized. They were there because they wanted to be there. The "A" school was still the draft. We had a lot of students that came and who really had no desire to be there. It took about six weeks to get them motivated. Once you got them motivated they learned very rapidly and did well.

The sad part was that some of the corpsmen would graduate and the next thing you knew they were the Fleet Marines over in Korea and a lot of them didn't come back. Once they graduated corps school they were sent with the Marines, or to other assignments. Education wise, they had what they needed, but did they have the experience? I think some of them didn't.

The corpsmen were sent to the front with the Marines. The corpsmen would stop the bleeding and then move the patient back to an area where they could be further stabilized. The medical care, like Commander Ruff (Ruff's War, 2005), is right up there on the front with the soldiers. They are doing the stabilizing. That used to be a job for the corpsmen. Now, the corpsmen put the wounded in a helicopter and bring them back to medical care, and during Korea we didn't have that many helicopters, though they were introduced during Korea. We had a helicopter pad aboard the hospital ship during World War II, but there weren't many helicopter patients coming.

In 1955, Alene went to Philadelphia Naval Hospital where she worked in the education department and in 1956 augmented from reserve status to regular Navy status. In 1958 she received orders to recruiting duty in Chicago and recruited in Wisconsin, Indiana, and Illinois.

In 1961 Alene was transferred to Subic Bay in the Philippines and ten months later to Yokosuka, Japan, as the assistant chief nurse and hospital detailer. It was also during this time that she was promoted to commander. The US was sending advisors to Vietnam during this period of time.

The USS Haven had been docked at Long Beach, California, as "the hospital" for active duty personnel. Alene received orders to serve in the clinics at that duty station from 1963 to 1964. In 1965 Alene reported in as senior nurse and instructor at San Diego Hospital Corps School.

We were very busy at that time. I think we had 10 to 12 nurses on the staff at corps school. They were trying to accelerate the program because of the need. Vietnam now was a shooting war. They needed corpsmen to go. I was there ten months when I got orders. I got a call from Captain Ruth Erickson, who was the director of the Navy Nurse Corps. She wanted me to come to Washington for an interview for a job that was going to be in the Pentagon. I went right away. The following day I was to go and meet with the assistant secretary of the defense for health and environment, Dr. Fisk. I figured that there would a group of us and we would each be interviewed. The job was to have something to do with recruiting. The sum and substance was that all the services—Army, Air Force and Navy— were having trouble getting sufficient nurses. The Army was sending nurses over to Vietnam right away. The assistant secretary of defense for health and environment was now going to assist with this because we were going to investigate whether we should change the requirements for recruiting. We were going to talk about how many people were coming, how many were needed and I was to be the liaison. No one had had that job before, so it was start from scratch. No one else was interviewed. I was it.

It was rather frightening. There was nothing to tell you exactly what you were to do, what was your job, what were the requirements, what was the goal. They told me to set up my goals and objectives and give it to them in ten weeks. I went back to San Diego and moved right away. I found an apartment in Washington close to the Pentagon. I was there a year.

They had not had nurse corps officers attached to the Department of Health and Environment. Now nurses are assigned there routinely. Dr. Fisk felt that we should recruit two-year graduates. He thought they could come in and do the job just as well as anyone else could, that all the services should open up to the associate degrees. I was very opposed to that. They could do the procedures and take care of the patients, but I didn't think they had enough experience. We were going to send them out into the MASH units, operating rooms, all these specialties and on ships. The big hang up was what were we going to call them? How were we going to rank them? What kind of rank would they get? Someone suggested they should be warrant officers. But they had already taken their state boards. They were already registered nurses. They were competing with the three-year nurses who had taken their boards and were registered nurses. The associate graduates said, "We are the same as the three-year nurses." The three-year nurses started as ensigns and if they had experience, sometimes they came in as JGs. The people who came in as JGs and lieutenants had at least bachelor's degrees.

The Army took in some of those associate degree nurses and I think the Air Force did. The Navy never did. We managed. We got through it okay without taking them in and going to the warrant officer. It wasn't too long before the other services dropped it because it was such a problem, as far as advancement was concerned. The warrant officer really isn't an officer. It is still an enlisted rank. We were trying to get the whole corps to have bachelor's degrees. We were trying to send a few active duty people back for their degrees. The ones who were being favored were the people who were active duty Navy, as opposed to reserves. The director of the Navy Nurse Corps was also opposed to accepting associate degree nurses.

Captain Erickson was replaced by Captain Bulshefski. She became the director of the Navy Nurse Corps while I was at the Pentagon. The Army took over the job I had at the Pentagon, a rotation-type job. Sometimes the Navy would have it, sometimes the Army or the Air Force. I went to the Bureau of Personnel (BUPERS) and I was the liaison between the Bureau of Medicine (BUMED), nursing division, and BUPERS. At that time the person who was doing the detailing was over in BUMED and didn't have access to any of the records. There was a set of cards with information on it and it was the only thing available to the detailer about people's assignments and rotations to different places. The nurse before me at BUPERS had access to the fitness reports. She could read what the person had done, about their assignments and educational backgrounds, so that we had some idea of where to place them. That was my assignment, to be that liaison between BUPERS and BUMED. I was in that position for a year.

I was reassigned to Great Lakes as the chief nurse. I think they are called director of nursing service now. It was 1968 and we were at the height of the Vietnam War. We were getting a lot of patients back from Vietnam. When I reported for duty they had 1,100 patients spread over a bunch of ramp-type wards. Of course, we still kept patients until they were able to go back to duty or were retired. We had so many orthopedic patients and amputees. We actually had an intensive care unit, but we didn't have any cardiac care unit. No one did. We had a recovery room attached to surgery; we started that unit. They used to all go back to the wards. If you had a private room, they would go there or they would go right up by the desk. Now people go into intensive care and then into progressive care units and then back to the ward. It is so common we don't even think about it, but we didn't used to have any recovery room or intensive care units. You went from the operating room to the ward and you were watched by the nurse right here by the desk.

Great Lakes had a lot of nurses, well over a hundred. I was very busy. One hundred nurses for 1,100 patients for three shifts is not a lot of nurses. However, we thought we were well staffed compared to some places. Of course, we had corpsmen and that was the big thing. I had some wonderful nurses. There were supervisors for certain areas and they really worked very hard. Unfortunately, a lot of them have passed away. A lot of them from that particular duty station have died. Almost all of them were younger than I.

In 1970, I was selected as the director of the United States Navy Nurse Corps. I had previously had a call to see if I would accept if I were selected, but I didn't tell anybody. I had been promoted to captain. I was up for promotion and I was pretty sure I would get that. I reported to the bureau in May and I relieved Captain Bulshefski. I was director from 1970 to 1975. That was a long time. There was a reason for that. Sign ups were one of our big things. We had nurses in Vietnam and nurses getting ready to go to Vietnam. You had to replace all of them here. Recruiting was slow. We weren't getting them in by droves. Jean Miller was the recruiter. Joan Engle, now Admiral Engle, was the junior recruiter.

It was a very busy time. We were trying to get people to school for their bachelor's and trying to send a few of them back for their master's. The emphasis was on the bachelor's. Then there were all the routine things in running the office. We had very busy days. I was not responsible for detailing the corps people. That was an enlisted thing. I was responsible for the nurses.

The thing I really wanted to do was to improve communication between people who were working in the hospitals and the Bureau. We each tended to do our own thing without communicating well with the other. You just didn't call the Bureau. You didn't talk to anyone in the Bureau unless it was an emergency. I made a lot of trips and visited a lot of hospitals and talked to people just to see what they wanted to do. I toured as many hospitals and clinics as I could.

I was at the Pentagon when they were working on Title 10 to open up promotions. Title 10 was signed and it allowed for more flag officers and this would allow all the other ranks to spread out and allow for more promotions. The people who had been lieutenants for ten years suddenly had the opportunity to become commanders, commanders to captains. We, the nurse corps, didn't have a flag at the top yet.

In 1970, right after I had been assigned to the Bureau, the Army promoted their first general, Anna Mae Hayes, the first woman general. That was the United States Army Nurse Corps. Five months later, General Westmoreland promoted the first line officer. Immediately after promoting General Hayes, the Air Force promoted their first woman general. That was a line officer, Jennie Holme. They promoted their first nurse corps almost at the same time to general. Then we waited. It didn't come through until 1972. I knew that someone was going to be promoted. I didn't know it would be nurse corps. I thought it would be a line officer. I thought they would dip down and choose someone that had previously been head of the Navy women. They were all highly qualified.

The American Nurses Association was meeting in Detroit in April 1972. I went to the Akron recruiting station and swore in a group of nurses in the late afternoon and I stayed overnight. Early the next morning I had a call from the Bureau from Jan Emil. She said, "They are asking for all kinds of information about you." It was BUPERS. I told her I was going to the convention. I am driving down the highway, on I–80, and I had the radio on and I heard I had been promoted to admiral. I was driving kind of fast because I was going to stop in Ohio and see my mother. This was a Friday afternoon and I was going to spend the weekend with her. I slowed down and it was about an hour when I went off the expressway and headed down the country roads. It was a toll road and I wondered as I went through the toll booth, "I wonder if that man knows what happened to me?" I was 52 years old at that time.

I drove to this little town in Ohio and my mother and stepfather came out to meet me, which was really unusual. My mother said, "Oh, I'm so glad you are home. The telephone is just ringing." The surgeon general had tried to call and all the admirals. The neighbors were there. The reporters were there. The reporter from Cleveland almost beat me home. There was all this publicity. It was unbelievable. About midnight they all left. In fact I had traveled in civilian clothes and when all these people were taking pictures my mother said, "You'd better go upstairs and put your uniform on." So, I did what my mother told me. It all quieted down.

I went on to Detroit. I was there two days and I decided I better go home. I had all these phone calls and I was getting calls from BUPERS to brief me because I was getting all these interviews. They wanted to brief me about Navy policy. If they had asked me about the Navy Nurse Corps, that would have been alright, but they weren't. They were asking me about Navy policy regarding women. No one else from the line was promoted. In fact, Maxine Conder, who followed me, had been promoted before the first woman Navy line officer.

The three years I was a flag officer were very busy years. We were doing recruiting. We tried to set up detailing with the qualifications you needed for each job. That was all just in its beginning at that time. Now it is all on computer. You say you need operating-room nurses? You need to know whether they can have change-of-duty orders and whether they were ready for change of duty. That all had to be taken into consideration. You couldn't just move someone from here to there because they had the right qualifications. You had to be sure you weren't moving them every couple of years. It was an expensive procedure. Jean Miller and Joan Engle never did have a computer. They did all of that longhand. They had lists of people who had qualifications. They had to find out whether they were eligible. They had to go to BUPERS and get the information. It was a long procedure.

I retired in 1975 at Fourth Street in Washington, D.C. That was in the Naval Yard. I had the whole thing. I had the band and the troops and everything. I had served for 32 and a half years. I watched nursing change from a job to a career, from a vocation to a profession, from good patient care to potentially miraculous patient care. It was an amazing experience. I was very grateful to have been part of it.

Merlan Owen Ellis

Many nurses serving their country during the Vietnam Era did not serve in Vietnam. Yet their contribution to the nursing profession and to the service members they served made a difference. Merlan Owen Ellis served during Vietnam, but not in Vietnam. His account reflects the changing times in the nursing profession, a time where men began to enter the profession of nursing and the area of expertise called "Public Health."

My primary academic interests centered in the biological sciences. By the summer of 1957 I had completed two years at Ricks College in Rexburg, Idaho, where I took as many courses in the biological sciences as time would permit.

I became intrigued with nursing as a potential occupation where the biological sciences could be combined with my newly acquired fascination with the behavioral sciences. I was totally unaware of the gender ramifications.

My father wanted me to inherit the family Idaho farm homesteaded by my grandfather in the late 1800s. I was his only child who could perform the labor-intensive farming tasks. When he learned I was considering nursing as a career, he was not impressed. He frequently encouraged me to "quit that nonsense, come home, and run the farm." Medicine or any other biological science would have been more acceptable. "Only women are nurses!" he would say. I learned he had great difficulty telling others about his son's choice for an occupation.

I wrote to the dean of nursing at Idaho State University (ISU) for information. She welcomed my inquiry and was anxious to have men as students in the school. The first and only man to have graduated from the school did so two years earlier. I was the second man to graduate for the ISU School of Nursing.

It was a challenge for a man to be a nursing student in the early 1960s. Some of the nursing faculty did not encourage a man in nursing, contrasted by full acceptance by physicians anxious to teach. For example, during my obstetrical rotation, my instructor would not permit physical contact with the mother except to massage her uterine fundus after the birth. It was an observation experience only, except for very understanding physicians who opened the back doors repeatedly. My obstetrical nursing instructor emphatically encouraged another course of study. I found her attitude quite puzzling. (As a rather amusing side note, when I took my state boards I received my highest score in obstetrics.)

The Army had a program for student nurses, fully funding the student's last two years of college. The student was on active duty assigned to the school with the pay grade of private first class until six months prior to graduation. The student then received an officer commission with the pay grade of first lieutenant with an active duty obligation of two years. As a husband with a child, this seemed to be an answer to prayers. However, men were excluded from the program! After loud outcries by other men and many women in nursing, the Army opened the door to men in the summer of 1963. I was accepted as one of the first men in the Army Student Nurse Program.

Historically, for centuries nurses were men. In the American Civil War both the Union and the Confederate armies had men assigned as nurses. At the turn of the century women in nursing started to organize. In 1894, the superintendents of female nursing schools (who were all female) gathered in New York City for their first annual meeting. The Nurses Association Alumnae of the United States and Canada had their first annual meeting in 1898. The delegates to their 1900 convention were reported to have only one married woman and no men. The Nurses Association Alumnae became the American Nurses Association (ANA) in 1917, and men were excluded until 1930.

One of the early accomplishments of the female nursing organizations was to exclude men from nursing in the military, partially as a result of the challenges women had as they sought acceptance by men, in this case, men in the military. Many women devoted years caring for military casualties and trumpeted the need for better care for these men without recognition.

In 1901 the Army Nurse Corps was formed where only women could serve as nurses. Many more decades passed before these female nurses received commissioned officer status. Men, during and prior to the Korean War, who were drafted or enlisted and were nurses, served in nonnursing capacities. Men were permitted to join the Army and Air Force Nurse Corps as commissioned officers in 1955, I believe partially as a spin-off from the women's liberation movements. It was another ten years before the Navy commissioned men who were nurses and admitted them into the Navy Nurse Corps. Another hurtle for men fell in 1963, when men were admitted into the Army Student Nurse Program.

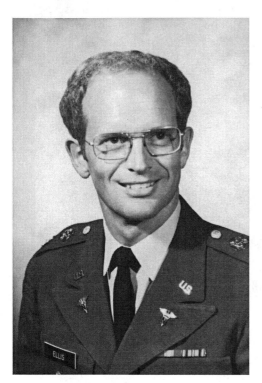

Merlan Owen Ellis at retirement.

In 1960 when the physician entered the charting area, nurses stood and the physician took the seat. The nurse did not speak unless the doctor spoke to her, a ridged rule for student nurses. Nurses were not permitted to do venous punctures. We took vital signs and felt fortunate to give routine injections. We sharpened needles on a whetstone prior to sterilization and reuse. It was an art to sharpen needles without creating curved barbs on the points. Almost everything was reused.

Many men who were nurses joined the military. In addition to better benefits than civilian nursing, the man was first an officer and then a nurse, which distanced him from social stereotypes.

After graduation in the fall of 1964, I went to Ft. Sam Houston (San Antonio), Texas for a two-month orientation to the Army Medical Department. The nursing section of the group was about one-third men from diploma and baccalaureate schools. It felt good to have male colleagues. However, a significant number of these men were privately homosexual, a preference totally foreign to this naïve Idaho potato farmer. To acknowledge their sexual preference would have resulted in an immediate discharge from the military.

Some of the male officers in other sections of the orientation group harbored the stereotypical image of men who were nurses. I remember one night the entire orientation group was in the field, each specialty tented together. It was a hot August Texas night; all tent flaps were raised. Loud sexual slanders were directed toward the tent with the male nurses for at least forty-five minutes. Comments were not reciprocated, only silence. Finally, with great relief, one of the instructors ordered the insulters to stop. This was my first personal exposure to intense prejudice, and it was to continue.

The nursing orientation included the various nursing specialties available in the Army. The student rotation I enjoyed most at Idaho State University was public health nursing. It was gratifying to work with public school students, provide guidance to families in their homes, and initiate needed preventive health measures. An application was submitted for an assignment in Army public health nursing, or community health nursing, as it was later called. There were about one hundred women in public health nursing in the Army at that time, but no men. The first three petitions to the Army Nurse Corps assignment branch in Washington were denied. After more communication between my advisor and assignments, I became the first man in public health nursing in the Army.

From San Antonio Merlan was sent to Fort Ord, California, for a year's internship in public health nursing, working with Henrietta Herman Pfeffer. Lieutenant Colonel Pfeffer was one of the first lieutenant colonels in the Army Nurse Corps, the highest rank in nursing at that time. She was the only community health nurse with the rank of lieutenant colonel.

I was assigned to Ft. Ord, California four months prior to an opening in the public health nursing internship. During that time I rotated through all patient care units in the hospital. The head nurse of the medical-surgical ward was a retired Army major who had served on active duty during World War II when men who were nurses were enlisted and not officers. She refused to call me "Lieutenant" even though the insignia was conspicuously worn on the uniform. She addressed me as "Sergeant."

The doctors had little experience working with men in nursing and had difficulty acknowledging me as a nurse. I was not addressed as "Lieutenant" but "Doc." The corpsmen were addressed as "Specialist," which corresponded with their rank. The doctors did not want to offend. They recognized the training and the contribution to patient care, but they just did not know quite how to relate to a man who was a nurse. I was independent as a public health nurse, doing assessments and bringing data back to the doctors as a colleague rather than the subservient role they assigned to hospital nurses. It was fascinating to experience the nurse/doctor relationship as it developed. The doctors eventually became comfortable with me as a nurse, in a male collegial sort of way.

The last rotation in the Ft. Ord Hospital was the emergency room, where I functioned as the head nurse. It was in that ER that I learned the value of the ward master, the senior enlisted person. I especially remember and appreciate one senior sergeant who took this neophyte officer under his wing and taught him the Army way. He would say, "Lieutenant, how about (this)?" When I made an administrative decision, he supported it almost without question. It was a great introduction to how officers and enlisted personnel function as a team.

There were no restrictions during the internship, even with mothers. Major tasks, assigned to me, included teaching new mothers how take care of themselves and their infants. Husbands were preoccupied with officer candidate school or other training in preparation for deployment to Vietnam. New mothers had little if any immediate or extended family support. Public health nurses attempted to fill the gaps by supporting these young mothers. The fathers, once they got over a man being the nurse, were very accepting and responded well to a man setting a parenting example for them. Trust and confidence developed. I was finally free to be a public health nurse. Being in homes with mothers and their children was not a concern.

Following the year at Fort Ord, I was transferred to Fort Belvoir, Virginia, fully oriented, fully expecting complete recognition and freedom to function. The greeting by the director and the other public health nurses who were all women reflected the same old quandary: A male public health nurse? What are we going to allow him to do? For the first year, I was not permitted to visit in most homes. My supervisor was more than willing to send me to visit the very elderly male retirees to change their catheters, but to be in a home with a new mother to reinforce breast and perineum care was not permitted.

The public health nursing section at Ft. Belvoir was designated a clinical training site for the Walter Reed Army Institute of Nursing (WRAIN). WRAIN was created to provide the increasing number of nurses needed by the Army Nurse Corps to fulfill its mission during the war in Vietnam. Students accepted to WRAIN received fully funded scholarships for their four years of college to include a military salary. A significant number of these students were men.

The public health nursing staff at Fort Belvoir was increased from four to ten with the charge to be ready to receive WRAIN students one year after I arrived. Each public health nurse was to have an expanded caseload of at least 40 families from which a broad range of experiences could be tailored for each WRAIN student. Since many WRAIN students about to arrive were men, the restrictions that remained on my practice had to be lifted.

The greater geography around the post was divided into public health nursing districts. My assigned area was south of Fort Belvoir in the Wood-bridge and Manassas, Virginia, communities. We nurses fine-tuned our newborn and infant assessment skills, focusing on normality and identifying what was not normal. Within a short period of time, we were independently holding in depth well-baby clinics. Ten of us assessed newborns from our respective geographical areas and fed the information to the one pediatrician in the clinic. He was very supportive. We found the clicks in the hips indicating possible congenital hip dysplasia. We found the heart murmurs and birth defects though we did not diagnose. We sent each child to the doctor for confirmation of our assessments and diagnosis. His most frequent feedback was "Good find." It was a wonderful collegial relationship. We, the nurses and doctor, had many discussions on topics of mutual interest, which greatly contributed to our knowledge base and confidence.

Many patients from my nursing district would receive services in a hospital clinic and then come to me for verification of the diagnosis and the care plan. In the mid–1960s private practice for nurses had not been conceived; however, we were essentially in private practice. We pioneered many areas of nursing, which was permitted under the broader Army umbrella.

During the late 1960s many military families were of the lower enlisted and officer ranks living off post with one or more children. For the junior officers, a family was considered a "luxury" not supported by the military. The officer could live in bachelor officer quarters but there was no place on post for his family. He received no additional financial support from the military if he lived off post with his family. The same was true for the lower-ranking enlisted soldiers. Many, both officer and enlisted, were living in extreme poverty given their low pay structure. Jobs for the wives were very hard to find and were mostly menial. The area was flooded with military personnel as a result of the buildup for Vietnam. Fort Belvoir was an enlisted training center with a large officer candidate school.

Nurses have historically been patient advocates, so as we became aware of the destitute situations facing these families, we felt something had to be done. We quantified hard data, which our director carried up through public health nursing command channels to the chief of the Army Nurse Corps and to the doctor over the Medical Department, the Army surgeon general. She was essentially told at each step that nothing could be done, to go home and to not be concerned. Such advocacy was not in her or our job description.

There is one attribute frequently given to public health nurses; they are very independent. Air Force personnel were also living with the same pay structure. The Air Force did not have public health nurses. With our encouragement, our director crossed services to the Air Force and again proceeded up through channels with the data. A little bit more empathy was given but the response was the same. The Navy was next. Again the data was taken through channels to top Naval officers who then crossed to the Army and Air Force commands and sought a combined effort to change the pay rates. As a result, there were eventually increases in the military pay structure up to at least the poverty level with family allowances. My wife and I would have had difficulty living on the local economy with two children on a first lieutenant's salary of $300 per month if my wife had not been an employed schoolteacher.

At Fort Belvoir I mentored many WRAIN students who were eager to learn public health. We worked with families, identified adults and children with medical deviations from normal, and advocated for their care. We assisted mothers with babies while dads were at war. We worked with the retiree population and their families and obtained hospice care and other services for them when needed. In addition while at Fort Belvoir I taught disease prevention to men and women in groups of 1,000 to 1,500 individuals as they completed their brief stateside training before heading to Vietnam. This learning environment was one of the highlights of my military career.

After Ft. Belvoir came an assignment to the University of North Carolina at Chapel Hill School of Public Health for a superb year of study for a master's degree in public health. There were 12 experienced international nurses in the public health nursing section, which made for a rich experience pool. Again, I was the only man. After graduate school came an assignment as the only military public health nurse in South Korea.

I wanted to go to Vietnam. I could see all sorts of public health activities that needed attention in Vietnam: venereal-disease awareness and prevention along with many other communicable diseases and health challenges. There were reports of 100 percent of companies with a venereal disease at the same time. I never assumed I would not go to Vietnam. I thought I would rotate there like everyone else but there were no public health nurses stationed in Vietnam. I supported the war, but in a different way: I helped sustain families of the men and some women who were in Vietnam.

The closest I got to Vietnam was South Korea. The assignment came immediately after graduate school. Primary tasks included disease investigation and prevention, services to mothers and infants (mostly Korean wives and girlfriends), school health for children of US personnel in Korea, inspection of health and dining facilities, and general community health.

Servicemen frequently fell in love with Korean women, married them, and had children or vice versa. A lot of these soldiers were quite immature with minimal education and experience. They now had a wife who spoke no English and usually a child. The social and cultural challenges for them were almost insurmountable. Helping the couple bridge the cultures and health practices was a monumental task.

Customarily when the Korean mother went home after delivering a baby, she would occupy the bed with the baby, father slept on the floor, and the Korean mother-in-law was in charge. The serviceman was expected to comply. I made home visits throughout South Korea to mothers and children to promote health. There were opportune times to also meet with servicemen as they faced family and cultural challenges. Travel to these homes was usually by jeep. Guards were left with the jeep. If a vehicle remained unguarded, it would be totally stripped by the time I returned.

Chaplains welcomed assistance as they counseled servicemen about to enter into matrimonial arrangements. Before the servicemen could get military permission to marry a Korean, they had to receive extensive counseling. My job was to introduce the potential wives to the American culture, a most challenging situation given the language barrier and women with no formal education.

If a Korean family had girls, the fathers were known to sell the girls into prostitution and slavery. The pimp would pay the family 200,000 wan for her. She was not freed from the pimp until she had earned an equal amount of wan and much more. Some of the girls did whatever was necessary to earn the money as quickly as possible. Some of them, whom I admired somewhat given their situation, desired a more acceptable lifestyle: They sought a serviceman with whom they could live all the time he was in Korea, or as long as he would have her, even if he had a wife in the States. The serviceman paid the pimp for her complete servitude without personal compensation. The Korean woman served the serviceman with intense devotion, interpreted by some men as love. The serviceman then reciprocated with a marriage proposal. Once a woman entered prostitution she was diminished to the lowest cultural stature. Marriage was a way to escape to a better life.

There were other servicemen, however, who used these women as slaves and treated them like slaves. I had the opportunity to offer assistance to some of these unfortunate women and counsel their keepers. They were ever so willing to please and to do anything they possibly could to stay with the serviceman even while being treated like something disposable. The serviceman might rotate to another assignment and leave the woman destined for a life of prostitution, an outcast from her culture. I have often wondered how these men, with these learned behaviors toward women, treated their wives when they returned to the States.

There was a ploy some of these women took. They willingly married the serviceman. As the couple was about to depart for the States, on a pre-planned schedule, their family would come rushing saying something like, "Your mother is dying. You have to stay." The wife would leave her husband on the tarmac promising to join him later but then never go to the States. He was married but without a wife and she had a military identification card with full military dependent benefits to include automatic pay deductions for wife support sent directly to the wife. Some women had multiple ID cards from previous marriages receiving wife support from all her husbands. She would buy items in the military exchanges that were hard to acquire in Korea and sell them on the black market. Trying to convince the serviceman, who thought he was in love and wanted to get married that this could happen to him, was a real challenge.

Many homes in Korea were heated with charcoal. The burning charcoal was outside next to an opening to an air flue that crisscrossed underneath the floor, heating it, and exited the other side of the building if everything worked well. Due to unsophisticated construction, noxious fumes frequently leaked into the house, resulting in carbon monoxide poisoning. Military rescue helicopters were dispatched to bring overcome individuals to our hyperbaric chamber. Some elderly men and women who were less sensitive to heat and who slept on the hot floor receive severe burns. Many of these patients were treated at the Army hospital. Service personnel were oriented to these dangers when they elected to live on the local economy with their Korean wives or girlfriends in her family home or in their own apartment.

The Korean culture is unique among Asian nations. There are fond memories of hiking through rice fields, visiting isolated silk factories and farming communities, enjoying the unique cuisine, and sitting on top of a mountain with a military radio listening to helicopter chatter in Vietnam. I will fondly remember my year in Korea and would like to have gone to Vietnam.

After the one-year assignment to Korea I was assigned as a member of the WRAIN faculty at Walter Reed Army Medical Center with a dual assignment to the University of Maryland School of Nursing as an assistant professor. Half of the 40-member WRAIN nursing faculty consisted of men. Members of the faculty were from 39 different graduate schools, which lead to some fascinating discussions as we attempted to define nursing as a unique profession. I was now one of the instructors who guided these gifted WRAIN students through didactic topics and accompanied them to their field experiences in my chosen profession of public health nursing.

_____

Merlan continued on in the Army Nurse Corps with his specialty in public health, eventually retiring from the corps after 21 years with the rank of lieutenant colonel and settling in Alaska.

Lois Gay

Lois Gay tells a story of the flight nurse during the Vietnam War. She tells it in great detail, helping the reader understand how important the flight nurse is during wartime. She also explains some of the emotional aspects of the Vietnam War not expressed in the same way by others.

I became a nurse because I watched my parents loving care for my brother, a cerebral palsy child, who was six years older than me. He could not walk or talk and had seizures most every day. As I got older, I realized the special care he needed and received. Having him at home taught us acceptance of those that are different and patience in caring for him unconditionally.

I graduated from Mercy Hospital School of Nursing in Altoona, Pennsylvania, in 1964 as a diploma nurse. Two classmates and I moved to Washington, D.C., and began work at George Washington University Hospital (GW). I wanted to work pediatrics, but GW didn't have a pediatrics department, so I worked on orthopedics. One of the nurses on my ward had just joined the Air Force and was being assigned to Washington state. I commented how neat that was. Her Air Force Recruiter called me that evening. He connected me with the nurse recruiter. I told her I wanted to work on pediatrics. She told me since the military at that time only had the operating room specialty for nurses, I would be signed in as a staff nurse. If my heart was set on pediatrics, the Air Force was not for me. If, however, I was willing to try, I would have a two-year commitment. The benefits were exceptional for a young nurse; 30 days of vacation annually, sick time if you needed it for however long it was necessary.

I took my oath in April 1965. Soon after that, my father became very ill and I left GW to return home to help my family. I talked to the recruiter and she put a hold on orders to become active. While at home, I worked at a school and hospital for retarded children where I thought maybe my brother could be placed.

That November my roommate from GW came home for Thanksgiving and had mail for me. She had not forwarded the mail since she was coming home. I had a letter welcoming me to Gunter Air Force Base, Montgomery, Alabama, for orientation and Maxwell Air Force Base as a new assignment. I was to report Jan. 6, 1966! I talked to a local recruiter and discussed the situation with my parents and left for the Air Force in Jan. 1966 with good wishes from all. They told me my brother was not my child and that I needed to try my wings and enjoy my career. My new job was on pediatrics! I was thrilled. My brother died unexpectedly Feb. 8, 1966, and my father died May 10, 1966, after a long illness. I used 21 days of annual leave that I had not yet earned, but I was happy where I was and made the best of it.

After a difficult year personally, I requested to go to flight nurse school and was granted that request as a first lieutenant. The slots were few and most always given to the highest ranking person applying. I was very fortunate! At that time those that finished flight school did not automatically get a flying assignment. Another surprise: I received a flying assignment out of Clark Air Force Base, Philippine Islands, when I finished flight school.

I reported to Clark Air Force Base, Philippines, in March 1967. I was 24 years old. The 902nd AES (air evacuation squadron) would be my home for the next 18 months. We flew in C–118s which had four propellers and could hold 20 liters of fuel and had 30 airline seats. We were equipped to give meds; oral, IM, IV, clean wounds and keep patients stable. Most patients were thrilled to see us because we were a big step to going home. The majority of the patients were amputees and gunshot wounds. Those on litters were in pajamas. Those walking were in uniform. It was always wonderful to get airborne because it was cool and the stench of the wounds was less.

We had four routine missions going to six different countries.

1. Clark Air Force Base, Philippines (AFB, PI), to Vietnam, deadheading (no patients). We spent the next 4 hours going to various bases along the coast of South Vietnam picking up patients. We would take patients to Cam Ranh Bay to the regional Army hospital and spend the night (RON). The next day was in-country Vietnam or a down day depending on the time we were returning to Clark.
2. Clark AFB, PI, to Vietnam, picking up patients and spend the night

101

at Cam Ranh Bay. The second day we would either deadhead or take Thai patients back to Thailand. We would stop at various bases in Thailand and move sick troops to Bangkok for treatment at the regional Army hospital. We would RON and then the 3rd day stop in Vietnam, pick up patients and take them to Clark.

3. Clark AFB, PI, to Korea. We would stop in Taiwan to refuel but Korean patients could not be off-loaded there, so it was just a brief stop. Once in Korea we had three places we could stop but we always ended at Osan AFB, Korea, for an RON. The second day we took American GIs that needed medical care to Japan. We flew to Tachikawa AFB, Japan. Third day we would do in-country missions in Japan and bring GIs or their dependents to Tachikawa for treatment or to deliver a baby. Fourth day we stopped at Kadena AFB, Okinawa, to off-load any patients returning from treatment in Japan. We would also pick up any patients needing treatment at Clark.

4. Clark AFB, PI, to Subic Bay, PI. We usually flew in a C–130 for this mission because it accommodated more patients and we went there to get patients from the hospital ships. It was only a half-hour flight but it was very hectic and we could give no meds or treatments. Our mission was to transport, but again, the morale was very high.

Special missions always originated at Clark for us. They may be initiated because we were told POWs (Prisoner of War) were being released near the Thailand/North Vietnamese Border or the Pueblo POWs (Korea) were going to be released. We would be dispatched to an area close to the release point and wait. We waited in four-day increments and then were replaced with another crew.

We usually had two nurses on a flight. Special missions may only have one. I was on such a mission in Thailand, which meant I had my own room. We were in a small town and a hotel with no security. I was scared to death. Our crew was like brothers to the nurses and I bunked in their room because I was afraid to be alone. They teased me but they understood and were very protective. Waiting is no easy thing but then again those we were waiting for had far more they were dealing with. I was on several special missions but never got to see the prisoners released.

I did go on a special mission to Iwo Jima, Japan, to pick up a patient who happened to be the medic assigned there. He broke his leg playing baseball. Before we left to get him we were given several bags of mail and

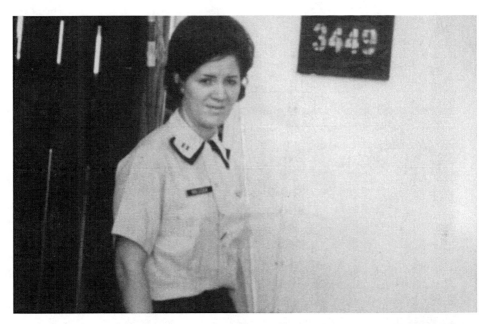

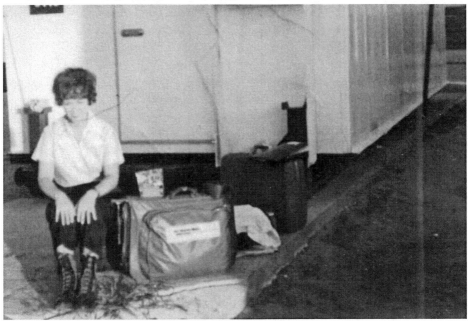

Captain Lois Gay, at nursing trailer, 1969 Cam Ranh Bay South, Vietnam.

some supplies and had the medic's replacement. They only got things by boat and that was not on a routine basis. We landed and the first thing I was asked was: "Do you need to use the latrine?" We had a "honey pot" (like an outhouse) on the C–130 which we flew in for that mission. I was going to say "no" but then said yes. Those assigned there got very little company and seldom a woman so they had cleaned the bathroom and put a "Women" sign up! Of course everybody knew where I went but they were happy I used it! I then got the patient and the first thing he said to me was, "Thanks for using the latrine!"

We had a special mission to Pleiku, Vietnam, to pick up Vietnamese POWs. It was more in-country and farther north than we usually went in our C–118s. We had a red cross on our tail but we did get fired on from time to time. Those on the ground brought the patients up the ramp to our door and our medical technicians took them from there. We were picking up three POWs. I was the charge nurse so the report was given to me and I inspected the patients as they arrived. The first one up was in position to be handed to our men and those carrying him dropped the litter! I was shocked and the pilot who was watching was just as shocked. The anger in the faces of those young GIs was eerie. The second patient was brought up by other litter bearers and they did the same thing. I wanted to scream at them but I couldn't even speak. The third patient was brought up and the transfer was as it should be. We got airborne as quickly as possible. Later, the pilot (a major) asked me why I did not reprimand the litter bearers. I replied that all I could think of was that we were there briefly to pick up the POWs and then gone. They were living much more stress day after day. It did not justify their actions but I did respect their situation and also that they were just kids doing the toughest job ever.

My last solo mission was in Thailand where I was staying in a hotel in Bangkok to relieve one of the nurse's stationed there. I had to lock my medical kit up at the squadron. During the night I woke up with a start! I had been bitten on the face by something and my face was swelling rapidly. I called the squadron and one of the medical techs came with medication to counter the reaction. He took me to the Army hospital for further treatment. I was grounded so could not fulfill my mission there and had to wait three days before I could return to flying. I also got a different room that I had sprayed for insects before I entered.

There were times when we would land at Clark in the late afternoon. The Air Force Band would come out and play music as the litters and ambulatory patients were off-loaded to welcome them closer to home! It was such a wonderful feeling to see everyone so happy. I thought I was very mature when I got to Clark but soon realized I was very naïve. The heartache of war took many forms, but realizing the majority of my patients were six to seven years younger than me was sometimes very difficult. Those that survived had so much to face once returning home with just physical problems not to mention the psychological injuries that might never heal. There was also much social stigma at that time. It was like leaving one war and dealing with an entirely different kind of war.

I was then assigned to Luke Air Force Base, Arizona, as a hospital nurse. It was quite an adjustment to be back to routine nursing in an older hospital. I had worked with all top notch folks, each with experience in the medical field as well as time in the Air Force. Now I was working with new med techs that had not been well taught or who were on their first assignment. I now had to regroup and face a different challenge. Most returning veterans didn't talk about the Vietnam conflict because it was so unpopular. They just wanted to get on with their lives. It seemed strange to get back into everyday life where we had all the comforts and everything we did was not daring and dangerous. Fitting back into a routine and finding a personal niche was very difficult for most everyone after that total experience.

In 1995 an Air Force nurse friend who was assigned in Vietnam while I was flying there, came to visit me at Bolling Air Force Base, Washington, D.C. She wanted to visit the Vietnam Wall. I had not been to see it. I just couldn't go there. We went together. It was a beautiful spring day and we got in a long line to walk by the wall. It was like going into a funeral home, the area was quiet and respectful. Many were touching and rubbing the wall. She recognized many names and "rubbed" a few. Since my contact with my patients was only a matter of hours on a flight, I didn't come to know anyone by name. My patients were the ones who survived. They either carried the hurt and injury silently or were the amputees and homeless in the streets.

The Vietnam Women's Memorial was dedicated in 1993. That event brought military nurses from all over the country together. I did not plan to attend at first because I only spent six years in the Air Force. Most of my friends remained in the Air Force and were lieutenant colonels or colonels. The day of the dedication we all gathered down by the Smithsonian's history museum. I saw the 902nd banner and met up with many that I flew with. Each of my friends went with their respective groups. We walked down Constitution Avenue with throngs of people on both sides of the street. We each got big hugs from "bikers" (Rolling Thunder) with the "Thank YOU Nurse!" It was wonderful to see more people there than listed on "The Wall."

We had a full weekend of remembering, crying, sharing and being truly thankful for this great country of ours. As nurses, we all talked about how young the men were and all those returning had so many challenges to face. We also discussed how we had each grown and all that we saw as young women. We were all serving in the military because we chose to, the men were drafted and had to serve. Even though many of us thought we were prepared for jobs, we had no idea all that it involved. We stuck together and helped each other as well. That bond has served us well.

I am writing these memories 44 years later. The aircraft is changed, the role of the flight nurse is different but as necessary. Sad to say, war continues. I'm happy to report that those who serve are recognized and appreciated for their service. Morale is high and that is the first step in a good recovery.

Sandra Kirkpatrick Holmes

This story demonstrates the difficulty of caring for patients in war time and the dedication of the nurses who do it. However, it also demonstrates that there is humor in the horrors of war.

As I look back and reflect, my career and many aspects of my life were quite serendipitous. I graduated from Nether Providence High School, in southeastern Pennsylvania in 1961 and was accepted at the University of Michigan. Going to Michigan was one of the first serendipitous events. The second occurred several years later, when I was looking for information about funding opportunities. On the bulletin board in the school of nursing there was a tear-off about the Army Nurse Corps Candidate Program. I called the Army recruiter. Anything I asked her was, "Of course you can," "Yes, the Army will send you to graduate school," "Being stationed in Europe is no problem at all," Anything I asked, the answer was "yes," which raised some issues and questions. It sounded too good to be true, and if it is you better look further.

Based on the advice of one of my professors, I contacted the Navy recruiter. The Navy had the same program as the Army. I applied and was selected. I came into the Navy Nurse Corps in July 1964, as a Navy Nurse Corps candidate. My tuition, books and fees were all paid by the Navy for my entire senior year. I received a small salary, which increased once I was commissioned as an officer, six months before graduation. In return, I owed them two years. When I got to pick where I wanted to go for duty, I had never been further west than Ann Arbor Michigan, so I put down all West Coast duty stations and received orders to the Naval Hospital, Oakland, California, also known as Oak Knoll.

I graduated from nursing school in May 1965, went to Newport, Rhode Island, for Officer Indoctrination School in August, and in September reported into Oakland. When I was asked where I would like to be assigned, I said pediatrics. They said, "No, think again." I had done my senior team leading on an orthopedic floor and I enjoyed that. So, I said orthopedics. They said, "Great. We need you on ortho."

Oakland was comprised of multiple single-story, wooden, barracks-type structures that had been built during World War II as temporary buildings. All of the wards and some clinics were connected by a series of wooden ramps and stairways. The orthopedic "ramp" or area consisted of four ortho wards, the urology ward and the ortho and urology clinics. Two wards or a ward and a clinic were connected by a much shorter "hallway" almost in the middle which formed an H. Each ward had 40 beds, 20 beds on either side. By the ramp there were two private rooms, the ward medical officer's office, the nurse's station and a treatment room. The utility room, the showers and heads (bathrooms) were all located in the middle connector section. Each building had a two-digit number and either an A or a B. One of the things that I constantly worried about was fire and evacuating the patients. Because those buildings were so old, I was told they would burn to the ground in less than five minutes! Very scary for a new grad.

When I first arrived at Oak Knoll, the ortho wards were all in the 40s and were located on the south side of the compound. Within a few days, we were relocated to 74A and 74B on the opposite side of the compound. A brand new hospital was going to be constructed right where the 40s ramp was located. I hadn't even received my state board results yet, but I was assigned to transport all of the narcotics from the narcotics locker on the ward that was closing to the new one. I got to the new ward with this bag full of narcotics, but nobody had the keys for the narcotic locker. We couldn't find the supervisor, so there I was hugging this brown shopping bag full of narcotics walking around thinking, "Oh my gosh, somebody's going to knock me off." Fortunately, I only had to "guard" the drugs for an hour or so and the rest of the move was uneventful. The lab, central sterile supply (CSR) and the orthopedic operating room remained close to where the former ortho wards had been. Our patients were transferred back and forth to the operating room in an ambulance. All of our bedridden patients were transported around the compound in an ambulance.

We didn't have crash carts. IV bottles, thermometers and syringes were all made of glass. Nurses had to match the number on the barrel of the syringe with the number on the plunger and keep them together with an elastic band before sending them to CSR for sterilization. Thermometers, suture sets, and glass syringes all had to be counted. If you didn't have a dirty one to turn in, you could not get a clean one without begging on bended knee. The 4×4s came in a great big loaf, and we had to make up our own smaller packages of 4×4s. We'd get the paper and tape from CSR and the bed patients could take half a dozen 4×4s, wrap, fold and tape the paper around them. It was good therapy. That was the, "You scratch my back, I'll scratch yours" kind of thing we often did between departments.

Another example involved the blood bank. Each unit of blood came with a pink tag which had three perforated sections so you could tear them off. One section was tied to the unit of blood. One was tied to the patient's bed or it went in the chart when the patient left the ward, and the third one stayed in the blood bank. The chief in the blood bank would send me a whole stack of pink tags and string and the bed patients would put the string through the holes in each section. Our patients often needed surgery several times a week and it was not uncommon to have four or five of them going to the OR each day. Since a type and crossmatch only lasted for 48 hours, it meant we had to type the patients really often. The chief would extend the expiration date an extra day until we got the hematocrits back. Then we could see how their crits were instead of having to go through type and crossing again. It was a trade-off.

One of my career highlights happened during my first tour of PMs. Admiral Nimitz was the only five-star admiral in the Navy at the time and there has not been another since then. He was a neurosurgery patient and had back surgery. Each shift one of the new ensigns was assigned to take care of him. I was called and told to report to the SOQ (sick officers' quarters) ward. I ended up caring for the admiral for my entire week of PMs.

One night I came back from dinner, checked in with the head nurse on SOQ to see if there was anything I needed to know, and she said, "No, but these flowers came for the admiral," as she pointed to a huge arrangement of anthuriums. Some people call it the little boy flower and you see a lot of them in Hawaii. They have heart-shaped leaves and red heart-shaped blooms surrounding a yellow pistil. I could see the card had the presidential seal. So I picked them up and went traipsing into the admiral's room and he promptly said, "Get those #@&* flowers out of here." I said, "But admiral, you didn't see who they're from." He said, "I said, get those #@&* flowers out of here." "But admiral, they are from the President of the United States." "I don't give a damn. Get those flowers out of here." Apparently this was one kind of flower he didn't like. So I took them back to the charge nurse and told her the admiral didn't want them and to give them to somebody else.

Shortly after that tour of PMs, my supervisor, Commander Jane Wathen, wanted to move me from the routine ortho ward to 76–B, the amputee ward. All the nurses on the ramp did change of shift report in her office, which was in 76–B. So I had walked through the ward every day and, as a brand new grad, it was absolutely intimidating. I didn't think I knew how to take care of those guys. It was difficult enough being on a regular ward. This was another one of my serendipitous events. Not only did I prove to be up to the challenge, I grew to adore working with those fellas and actually looked forward to going to work each day.

It was a handful though. We had four or five surgeries every day. We had to mix our own IVs. They weren't done in the pharmacy. At one point, we had so many really ill patients that CDR Wathen would try to assign one extra nurse who did nothing but mix IVs for the next 24 hours, just for 76–B. On the 3 to 11 shift there were usually two corpsmen on each ward and each nurse covered two wards.

On AMs there were two, maybe three nurses and two to three corpsmen. Every patient got a bath and clean sheets. We always had patients who were running fevers of 102 or 103. Because they were wounded in a filthy environment (like rice paddies fertilized with human waste) almost every wound was infected with pseudomonas. The sickest patients and the ones who were running the highest fevers were in the two beds adjacent to the nurses' station. The wards were not air conditioned. In the summer we had these huge floor fans that were probably two or three feet in diameter on pedestals and they were put next to the first two beds. Whatever germs the patients had were being blown all over the ward. If we weren't sure what was causing their infections, we put a stainless steel basin containing Betadine and hot water on an overbed table at the foot of their bed. The instruments from dressing changes, their plates, silverware, etc., were all put in the basin. If we were lucky, it got changed once a day and that was our infection control. Things have really changed since then.

I hadn't been on the amputee ward at Oakland very long when California Governor Brown came to visit on Veterans Day, November 1965. It seemed like every dignitary who came to the hospital wanted to visit the Marine amputees on 76–B. Captain Bulshefski, the chief nurse, came up to the ward that morning while I was frantically trying to get everybody's baths and A.M. care done before the governor's expected arrival between 0900 and 0930. She walked down the ward and lowered all of the Venetian blinds to the same level. Then she turned all the wheels at the foot of the beds in same direction. She put pillowcases on the pillows on the empty beds. It was really kind of neat that she didn't tell me to get this done, she just did it herself. They were things I would never have worried about or fooled with, even for the ward inspections on Fridays. Perhaps it was an old Navy or nursing school habit.

My first tour of nights was over Christmas, December 1965. We did 14 straight nights. We covered the five wards on the ramp; four ortho wards, one urology and we were also on call and standby for the urology and ortho clinics. There was one corpsman on each ward. So, you were really hopping as the acuity and the number of casualties increased.

Because of the staffing on nights, the 3 to 11 shift tried to give all the patients their sleeping pill, pain medication and can of beer. Most of them had an order for a can of beer. Almost all of them had lost weight and looked so terribly thin and skinny. The beer helped them put some weight on and it also helped them sleep. So we made a real effort to work with them and hold off the pain medications as long as we could, then medicate everyone close to 1030 or 1100. That would give the night nurse time to check the other four wards and then get back to the amputee ward, which was the busiest with the most acute patients.

I don't think I realized at the time, but while I was giving physical bedside care, I had actually woven psychological patient support into that as well. I could be caring for one patient, but be carrying on a conversation with several of them all at the same time. Over the years, I have spoken with many amputees and health-care providers and we all agree that the open-bay wards were the best way to provide patient care and psychosocial support for the amputees as well. I was used to the open-bay ward from my student days at the University of Michigan. I think there is room for both open-bay and closed-room type of situations. There are times when patients need their privacy and there are times when those open-bay wards were just wonderful.

The sickest patients were closest to the nurses' station at one end of the ward. The three to four at the opposite end were the ones closest to discharge. We actually rearranged the beds with the guys in them on a daily basis according to acuity. We usually received casualties two to three times a week. In 1965, there were no hospital ships, no Navy nurses in Vietnam. Casualties were initially treated in 'Nam, flown to the Philippines or Japan and then on to us. Fellows who were on their "pity pots," feeling sorry for themselves, could look to either end of the unit. At one end was someone in worse shape than they were. Those who were ready to be discharged could look the other way and see that they had come a long ways toward recovery. They could see that there was someone worse off. Being a Marine is the epitome of *esprit de corps*. They all pitched in and helped one another.

One of my favorite "sea stories" involved one of my first inspections on 76−B. Every Friday morning there was command inspection. Every ward, clinic and space in the hospital was inspected. Every drawer had to be open, every patient bedside locker had to be open and its contents neatly organized. No "gear adrift" and no civilian clothes were allowed on the ward. In the linen room everything had to be stacked just so. I was standing in the middle of the ward at 0959 with a wheelchair loaded with hangers, coffee mugs, civilian clothes and all sorts of gear adrift and absolutely no place to put any of it. One of the patients said, "Here Miss K., we'll fix it for you. Just give me this stuff." I said, "Okay, fine," left him with the wheelchair and went to the ward entrance to meet the inspecting officer. As I escorted him through the ward, I noticed the wheelchair, but there wasn't anything in it. I looked around and the guys are just grinning. Then, I noticed that the bilateral amputees had all grown legs. One leg might have been all the coffee mugs, another leg the clothes, etc. That became our practice every Friday. They would just take it all and make it look like legs. They were a very creative group.

As a disciplinary measure, one of the nurses took away one of the patient's wheelchairs. She put it in the sun room at the far end of the ward. The patient was a bilateral amputee who was bound and determined to get it. He used the balkan frame on each bed to swing from one bed to another all the way down the ward to reclaim his wheelchair. Where there was a will, there was a way. While these antics were humorous, psychologically they were also very healthy and healing for the amputees.

I learned a lot from these men. You have to remember that there were maybe four to five years difference in age between me and most of them. I was naïve and innocent. I was helping a patient with his bath one day. I said, "You have the most unusual freckles I have ever seen. I have never seen anyone with gray freckles." He said, "Those are powder burns." I was so embarrassed.

One day during morning rounds or sick call, we had already seen about three quarters of the patients when we came to Ray's bedside. While he wasn't an amputee, he was on 76−B because his wound was badly infected.

He had a gunshot wound to his elbow and that arm was in a Statue of Liberty cast but he never complained. Usually very glib and talkative, this time he was hemming and hawing, he kept saying, "I um, I um." So I said, "Come on Ray, what can we help you with?" "Well, I um, I um." After a few minutes of this, I finally said, "Listen Ray, we don't have all day. Doc Salisbury has to get to the OR. If you have a problem, spit it out. We're here to help you." He said, "I have crabs." I immediately replied, "Where are they? I'll take them home and cook um." Needless to say, the entire ward erupted in laughter. Dr. Salisbury looked at me and shook his head, finished sick call, then took me into his office where he drew this little oval with lines off either side. He said, "What does that look like?" I said, "It looks like some kind of little bug." "It is *pediculus pubis*." "I know what that is. It's lice." "Well, the guys call it 'crabs.' " I was mortified. Of course, from then on the fellas teased me unmercifully. Each morning for a while, when I walked on the ward some one would hold up his thumb and forefinger pinched together and say, "Miss K, I've got some crabs. Want some?" Talk about total innocence.

One amputee who was in the Army and had been drafted, didn't want to go to physical therapy. He just wanted to stay in bed and vegetate. He was uncooperative, kept to himself, had no visitors and made no effort to talk to any of the other patients. Needless to say, caring for him became extremely frustrating as well as challenging. CDR Wathen said, "You know, the only thing you can do is throw a pitcher of cold water in his face, and that is perfectly acceptable." We only had to do that a couple of times and he started to shape up. Treating a patient that way as a brand new graduate was terribly hard. The fellows taught me tough love and I can say, after 26 years, it was really and truly a gift from them.

I received orders to Guam in 1967. I was there from June 1967 until December 1968. I was the charge nurse on one of the two orthopedic wards. We had 40 beds in the main ward, but the "sun porch" had 20 bunk beds. So it was possible to have a census of 80 at any given time. We either treated the casualties and returned them to duty in 'Nam or stabilized them for medevac back to the States. Sending the fellas we had treated and cared for back to Vietnam was one of the toughest things we had to face. We knew the odds. We knew what awaited them and so did they. It was equally difficult when the young corpsman we had worked so closely with received orders to the Fleet Marine Force, which meant Vietnam. That was truly devastating because corpsmen had one of the lowest survival rates.

I keep in touch with more people from that duty station than any other. No doubt it is because of what we went through together, what we endured and indeed survived. We were there during the Khe Sanh and the Tet Offensive in 1968. During Tet, medevac flights with casualties arrived every single day rather than three times a week. Not only were we overwhelmed by the numbers, the casualties were really in bad shape. They would be stabilized in Vietnam and then sent on their way. It was an extremely hectic time clinically with the medevacs. Everybody you worked with, the doctors, nurses and the corpsmen, knew what you were up against because we were all in the same boat. It wasn't easy for any of us. Thank goodness for the Serenity Prayer. It became my mantra during the darkest days.

Our OR schedule was single spaced, on both sides of a legal piece of paper. We would do two cases in one room at a time with one nurse anesthetist or anesthesiologist for both patients. We even opened an annex hospital known as Asan. We had to expand. ICU, ortho and medicine stayed at the main hospital and the annex was mainly for general surgery patients. Additional doctors were even assigned from the States for temporary additional duty, or TAD.

One of the differences between the Army and the Navy Nurse Corps policies during Vietnam was that Captain Bulshefski, director of the corps, was adamant that nurses, particularly new graduates, not go overseas, not go to Da Nang, not go to one of the hospital ships unless they had a full, two-year tour stateside first. She wanted them to have that tour at one of the large Navy teaching hospitals where they would get some experience with casualties. She wanted them to get out of school, go through Newport, get clinical skills established, and get used to the military. The Army didn't do that. Frequently, Vietnam was the first duty station for many of their new graduates. I always felt that the nurses in-country (Vietnam) had it worse than we did because they dealt with so much death and dying. I didn't lose any patients on Guam on the orthopedic ward and only two at Oakland. However, those who served in-country felt that they didn't have to deal with any of the families. Nor did they have to deal with any of the psychosocial aspects of rehab and returning to the civilian world. And that was no doubt very true.

There were some memorable patients on Guam. Ted, a Marine amputee, talked to me for hours about the war during a tour of night duty. The day he was medevaced back home, he gave me a lighter that was engraved: "To Miss K from all the guys shot up in the dirty little war." I cherish that. Then there was Tim Davis and Bill Gostlin. Tim was severely wounded, lost both legs above the knee and spent several days in ICU before he came to my ward. Bill had lost one leg below the knee. They served together in 'Nam and were in beds side by side directly across from the nurse's station, which was in the center of the ward. They would repeatedly pull pranks on one another and seemed to play a game to see which one could get their next pain medication first. Tim was finally well enough to go to the movie one evening. However, in the process of transferring from his bed to the wheelchair—it was one of the really old-fashioned, high-back, caned ones—he ended up sitting on the floor instead of in the chair. One of the things I had learned by "my guys" at Oakland was tough love. They must learn to help themselves. You can't mollycoddle them. The air turned blue when I told Tim to act like a Marine or I would not help him. If he was well enough to go to the flick, he was well enough and strong enough without legs to get up into the wheelchair by himself. It took him about 15 or 20 minutes, but he managed. The entire ward applauded and he went triumphantly off to the movie. It would be more than 25 years before I knew the impact I had had on these two fellas.

Toward the end of my tour on Guam, I was still single, and with a little encouragement, decided to extend in the Navy for another tour of duty. I requested Bremerton, WA, recruiting in San Francisco, or Camp Pendleton, CA. I received orders to the Naval Hospital on the Marine Corps Base, Camp Pendleton, and worked on the orthopedic ward there. The day my household goods were delivered to a cute little house I was renting, and the movers had left, I sat down to decide what kind of curtains I was going to make. The phone rang and it was Bess Feeney, the chief nurse. She said, "How would you like to go to recruiting duty in San Francisco?" I said, "Well, I did put that on my dream sheet. But they just delivered my household goods." "Oh, they'll move you again. Come to my office tomorrow, we'll call the recruiter and find out what recruiting duty is all about." I was only at Pendleton for the first four months of 1969. I unpacked just enough to be comfortable.

It was the first time I had ever worked with Marine Corps recruits. They had to request permission to speak before they asked for anything. You didn't want to undermine their training. It could be a fairly busy ward at times, especially on evenings when medevac casualties arrived. One night when I got home from a tour of PMs, I realized, "I've seen enough of this. It really is time for me to go." I had admitted a youngster with multiple shrapnel wounds to both legs, relatively minor injuries compared to all of my amputees. For some reason, he got to me and I was glad I was going to have a break from bedside nursing and Vietnam casualties. While there I worked with some nurses who had been stationed in Da Nang. The chow carts were pulled to the wards by little mini tractors and we could hear them coming down the ramp. It was really scary for one of the gals who told me that they sounded exactly like incoming in Vietnam.

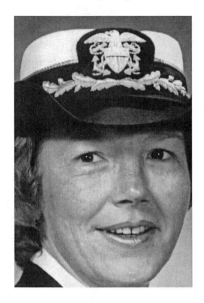

Sandra Kirkpatrick Holmes on active duty.

After four months I was off to recruiting in San Francisco. It is the only time I lived downtown in a city. My office was in the Federal Building, which had been Admiral Nimitz's headquarters during WW II. It was located near Market Street and the opera house. I covered two thirds of California, Nevada, Utah and Hawaii. I would go to Hawaii once a year to attend the state nurses' convention. Some of the schools in California were a good five-hour drive from my office. Antiwar sentiment was very high. I was even threatened once in San Francisco. A hippie-type called me a killer. I pointed to the oak leaf insignia on my sleeve and said, "I'm a nurse. I don't even know how to handle a gun. I put the bits and pieces of America back together." I used public transportation to go back and forth to work because parking downtown was a hassle. After the hippie incident, I asked the commanding officer's permission to wear a civilian raincoat over my uniform. Several of my patients had told me that feces was thrown at them or their medevac buses en route to Oak Knoll. It was difficult, but I don't recall anything negative or a lot of antiwar activity at the schools of nursing I visited. Many of them were in the heartland, farmland away from San Francisco and Berkley—the hotbeds.

As far as I can tell, I never experienced post-traumatic stress, probably because I stayed in the military, wrote about my experiences and did a tremendous amount of public speaking while on recruiting duty. All of this allowed me to vent about all of my experiences and how difficult it had been. Interestingly, every time I spoke, I was asked, "Wasn't it depressing?" I would always respond, "No, it really wasn't. These fellows would get their prosthesis. They could get up and walk and do everything and anything that you and I can do. Compare that to a pediatric ward with little ones with leukemia or a Wilms' tumor or visit the neurosurgery ward with the paraplegics and quadriplegics, as well as the ones with severe brain damage. To me caring for them would be awfully depressing. Being with the amputees wasn't depressing. It was and honor and a privilege to work with them. They were my heroes. I received as much if not more from them as they received from me in terms of growth. Not only did I learn tough love, but also

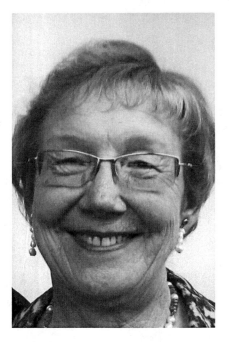

Sandra Kirkpatrick Holmes, 2012.

that there is always somebody in worse shape than you are. Life is good.

Sandy continued her Naval career until retiring as a captain in June 1990 with a total of 26 years of active duty service. She described her experiences with amputees in two articles. "Battle Casualty: Amputee" was published in the American Journal of Nursing in May 1968 followed by "Hey, Hero!" in the Reader's Digest *in September 1970.*

Her story doesn't end here. In 1993 the nurses who were stationed in Guam with her decided to have a 25th reunion. The planners chose Washington, D.C., and the November weekend coinciding with the dedication of the Vietnam Women's Memorial.

I had been stationed in Washington for five years and did not plan to attend the reunion. But a friend wrote a note encouraging me to come and be her roommate. Reluctantly I agreed. Little did I know that it would be another serendipitous event in my life. Saturday late afternoon, following the parade and dedication ceremony, my friend and I met up again in our hotel room. We hadn't seen each other all day because she was one of the state co-chairs for Virginia and was in VIP seating. She asked me as we were watching the news and coverage of the ceremony, "Do you remember a patient named Tim Davis or a Bill Goslin from Guam?" "I cared for three amputees named Davis," I replied. Tim somehow saw my friend's name badge with "Guam 1968" on it and had asked her if she knew a nurse named "Miss K." Long story short, we met the next day on the steps of the Lincoln Memorial. Tim had been looking for me since he read my article in the *Reader's Digest*. According to him, the incident with the wheelchair, "Saved my life. It turned my life around. I was ready to give up. I thought that without legs my life was over." With a twinkle in his eye he insisted on showing me how he can now get back into his wheelchair in only 5 seconds. "When I help as a counselor at the wheelchair camp for kids, this is one of the drills I make the kids do every day," he said triumphantly.

Bill appreciated being pushed to go to PT because he was always full of excuses. He gave me his Purple Heart. "I was going to leave this at the Wall. But you deserve to have it," he said. I felt so humbled when he gave it to me. I was just doing my job and I know that must sound mundane, but I loved what I was doing. I was hoping and praying I'd make a difference ... something a little better out of the horror of Vietnam. There aren't words to describe the feeling that I had knowing that I had made an impact. Most folks live out their lives and never know if they have had a positive effect on another human being. For years I had wondered "Why me? Why amputees?" On the steps of the Lincoln Memorial in 1993 those questions were finally answered.

Lynn Calmes Kohl

Lynn Calmes Kohl's story is one struggle, of real concerns about the situations she found herself in and the consequences of her experiences. She gives details of recruitment and service that were not common to many other nurses, but were very real.

I enrolled in nursing school immediately after high school in 1965. I lived in Appleton, Wisconsin, and attended Mount Sinai Hospital School of Nursing in Milwaukee. It was a three-year program. In the spring of 1968, during my senior year, I heard about the opportunities connected with being in military service. The recruiter told us because we were graduates we would become officers. We could also get our choice of duty stations. He proceeded to tell us about Fort Ord and how it was right by the California beach. I later found out the hard way that Fort Ord was the staging area for nurses to be sent to Vietnam.

I had friends, both males and females, who had just come back from Vietnam. They advised me not to go to Vietnam. So I had these reservations and talked to the recruiter about it and he told me that there was no way a female could be sent to Vietnam unless she volunteered. If a female volunteered she would be sent there in a week because there was a shortage of nurses. I then went back and thought about it. Everyone else was excited about it. Fort Ord at the beach sounded really good. None of us had any other commitments. The recruiter called to tell us that a group of Army men were going on maneuvers down to Florida the next weekend and asked if we wanted to come along. That sounded great to us, thinking that we were going to be with a plane full of guys.

They wined and dined us. We thought that was pretty neat and that we should try it out for a while. The other girls signed up right away. I still had reservations so I talked to the recruiter again and he again insisted that there was no way that the Army would send a female to Vietnam unless she signed up to go. For about a month or so I was indecisive. I went back to talk to him a couple more times and every time he said the same thing. Finally I joined.

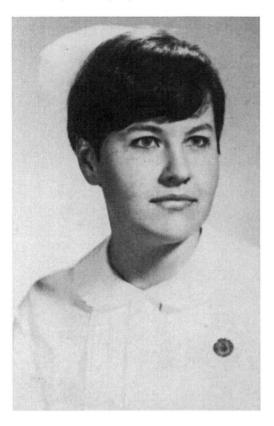

Lynn Calmes Kohl, 1968 graduate of Mt. Sinai Hospital School of Nursing.

For three months during the summer I worked in post-operative nursing. When fall arrived, the four of us girls went to Fort Sam Houston for basic training. When we received orders for Fort Ord, we were very excited. We arrived there on January 1 and I was placed in pediatrics. Less than a month later I received orders for Vietnam. I explained to my commanding officer that I had been told that I would not get orders to Vietnam unless I signed up to go. She asked if I had that promise in writing. Within a month all the other girls had their orders for Vietnam, too. The girl who had talked us into joining the service went AWOL, got pregnant and was out of the service. The remaining three of us were sent to sunny Vietnam.

On the flight over there was dead silence, nobody talked. Everyone was absorbed in their own thoughts. When we arrived in Vietnam, we flew into Nha Trang. It was kind of late in the day, so we spent the night there. All the nurses were placed in the female military barracks. As we stepped off the plane the heat and the smell were overwhelming. It was an unpleasant, unusual smell. It kind of hit me and caused me to stop for a second to absorb what was going on around me. All of a sudden I heard a pop. People were running toward us and pushing us down the steps telling us to run over to a building because we were under small arms attack. It became very apparent to us that we were under small arms fire and that this was for real!

120

We went to the nurses quarters in Nha Trang. The next morning a friend and I went to get our assignments, still thinking that we were going to be stationed together. We were sent to two separate places. She went north. I was sent to the 71st Evacuation Hospital, Pleiku, in the Central Highlands. She left earlier and there were two choppers that took off. The first one took off and we then followed. The chopper ahead of us was shot down. I watched it as it fell.

When we got to Pleiku, it was too late in the day to get our orders. They took me to my hooch and I met my hoochmates. We had a sidewalk outside our hooch on a big hill with a big red cross. We were all sitting outside during the evening and all of a sudden I heard a whistle and a thud. I then

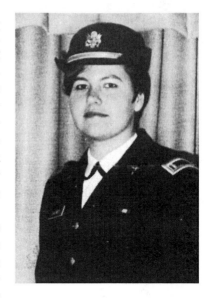

Lynn Calmes Kohl in dress blue uniform.

looked around and realized that I was by myself. There had been about six or seven people sitting around just a second ago and I didn't know where they had gone. Suddenly one of my hoochmates appeared and pulled me inside. She told me to crawl under a bed and stay there until she came to get me. We were under a rocket attack!

We named Pleiku "Rocket City" because we were under rocket fire almost daily. I would wake up in the morning under my bed and realize that we had gotten hit again. After a short period of time I didn't think I'd survive so I sent my will to a friend in Milwaukee. I came to that conclusion right after those rocket attacks. The corpsmen were upset that we didn't have bunkers around our hootch so they brought sand bags and made an embankment around it. This provided something to at least block some of the incoming shrapnel. That was all we had.

We were under attack one night and the compound was overrun. The next morning I opened the door and there was a dead NVA (North Vietnamese Army). Had he survived and gone through the door, he would have killed me. I was in the first room through the door. The women didn't get to carry guns. We didn't even get combat pay. There were bunkers for the male officers and enlisted men, but not for the nurses. All the enlisted,

121

male nurses and doctors carried guns, but not the female nurses. When we went through the MOC village during our training for Vietnam, we only walked through the "jungle." We sat down on the bleachers and we were handed a gun which we were only allowed to look at. We were not allowed to fire it because we were females.

The next morning I went to get my duty orders. My MOS was post-op nursing because I worked three whole months in that unit stateside. So I thought that I was going to post-op. They told me I had to go to surgery. That, in itself, was traumatic as I'd had a very bad experience in the OR in nursing school. The requirements to work in the OR in a combat zone included either completion of their one-year OR combat training program or three years civilian nursing experience in the OR. I had neither. But they needed somebody, so I was ordered there. When I arrived to the unit, the head nurse told me that they had many bad cases going on. She told me to mask and gown and she assigned me to a case and told me to stand there and observe. I was going to start as a circulating nurse and later proceed to scrubbing.

I was gowned and masked and assigned to a young man who had already received 100 units of blood. He had lost a leg and his one arm was hanging by a tendon. He had abdominal wounds. As I observed, one of the doctors looked up and became very angry because I wasn't doing anything. He threw the scissors at me and yelled for me to cut off the arm. My first five minutes there I had to cut an arm off. After that it was downhill all the way!

There were big helicopters, Chinooks, that held a hundred or more patients. I may have just finished a shift and would be walking back to my hooch. On seeing one of those helicopters headed for our hospital, I would turn around and head back to the OR. I would be in the OR for days. We stayed until the last patient was gone. During those pushes there weren't enough doctors and nurses, so the nurses and corpsmen had to do the minor surgeries like debridement. We all had to perform each other's jobs. Because of this I was always concerned that someone wasn't walking because of me. Maybe I could have cut a nerve or a tendon and because of that the patient couldn't walk. I questioned if we did more harm than good. The doctors showed us what to do only once and then we were on our own. I wasn't prepared to do that.

I never looked at names. I had to write them down but I didn't want to remember them. Another hard part was that the men were sent to us

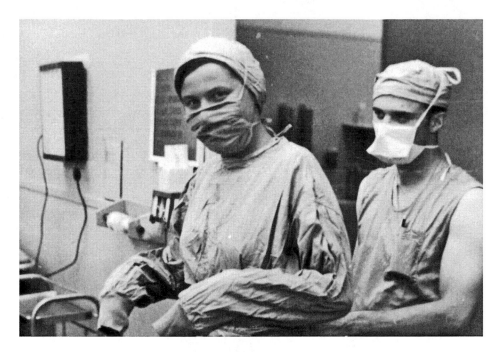

Lynn, gowning and masking for OR case.

directly from the battlefield. They went to surgery and post-op and when stabilized enough they were sent to Cam Ranh Bay or Saigon. From there they became more stable and went to Japan or Guam and then back to the States. We didn't know who died or survived. There was no way to know. That was very hard, not knowing if all our hard work was in vain or not.

I helped deliver a baby of a Vietnamese woman. We were able to treat her because her husband was an officer in the South Vietnamese Army. When she arrived, she was very stoic. She did not look like she was in any pain. She did not make any noises and was very quiet. So we thought that she was in the first stages of labor. I was told to sit with her for a while. All of a sudden she made the smallest noise. Something told me that I had better look and I took the sheet up and there was the baby crowning. So, I delivered it. The baby and mom turned out okay. That was one of the few positive moments over there.

Outside of the hospital there was a MARS unit, the Special Forces camp and an Air Force base. We were there for the 4th Infantry Division which was not very far from us either. I kept running into one of the men from the Special Forces who had a jeep and one evening he asked me to go out for a ride with him. I agreed only if my friend would come along. So we all went out. It was at night and we went out of the compound. It had just rained so we were hitting puddles and the mud was splashing up all over us. I was wearing a bright orange dress. We were drenched in mud and laughing. The next morning I woke up wondering why I went out the previous night. It was in the middle of the night and the NVA were out there and there were mines everywhere. I had on a bright orange dress. That was a perfect target. I never did anything like that again.

Since it was safer for us to stay in the compound, the swimming pool was a source of recreation. We could only go in the swimming pool if there was a life-guard present. The lifeguards were the corpsmen. They not only worked the same hours we did but also worked guard duty. There was an instance when we were under rocket attack while we were in the pool. There was a person who basically crossed the pool walking on water. I never saw anyone move so fast in my life!

Through all these experiences I built a wall to block my emotions and as a result I find myself expressing my emotions inappropriately. There is anger deep inside of me. I am angry at everything. Because of this I take counseling with a men's group. They're the same men that were in the group when I started it many years ago. They are still talking about the same things and they've not moved on. I spent three years in a women's group in Minnesota and we moved on. We progressed. Unfortunately all my appointments had been cancelled due to budget cuts. The men's counseling group can only meet once a month for an hour. That is not enough time to accomplish anything.

I was asked to give a Memorial Day speech. I focused on how people need to look at the consequences of war and that there's more to war than going overseas and kicking butt. There are lifetime consequences. The day we left Vietnam we thought that the war was over but a few years ago we went back to Vietnam on a healing journey and people are still suffering from the consequences of the war. While we were there, we discovered that there are over 5,000 babies born with the aftereffects of Agent Orange. Each year people are still stepping on land mines and are either being killed or maimed. The Vietnam War ended in 1975 but for them the war continues. Most of them are Buddhists and they believe that the past is the past and they are living in the present. They recognize that those of us who were over there had to do it because it was our job. Now they welcome us. It was really healing to be accepted by them.

Our tour group was the first one to return to Pleiku. From talking to the guide I found out that the hospital I had worked at became the largest and best hospital of the Central Highlands. I felt really good that people didn't run off with everything and dismantle the hospital. Everything was left there. Usually the Vietnamese would strip a place once the Americans abandoned it. We went to the different camps where the men were and there we found bare land and some sand bag pieces sticking out of the dirt. That was all there was left.

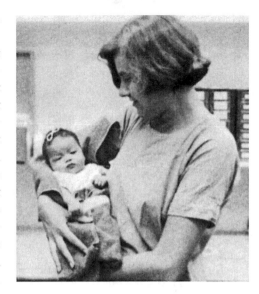

Lynn, with baby delivered in Vietnam in 1968.

My parents never had a vacation so for their wedding anniversary I sent some money to a friend in Milwaukee to get tickets for my parents to fly to Hawaii. Their anniversary was about the time I was ready to leave Vietnam. I got the delay en route to go there before I went home. So all year I saved my money. We were going to stay at the best hotels and we were going to island hop. It was going to be the best vacation they ever had.

When we got to Vietnam, we had to change our money into MPCs, which we called "funny money." Two or three days before we would leave we would get it changed back. All the money I saved I turned over to get back American money. I was still working a couple days and kept it in the pockets of my uniform. I even slept with the money in my pockets. The afternoon that I was leaving I still had to work in the morning. I changed my uniform from the one I had slept in to a clean uniform. I had just taken the pants off and the girl down the hall screamed, so I went running down to see what the problem was. Next thing I knew I saw our mamasan running out of the hooch really fast. I just knew what had happened. When I returned to my room, sure enough, all my money was gone. I quickly put on another pair of pants and went chasing after her. We screamed to the

MPs to stop her but they didn't understand what was going on. The girl ran right past them. I had told my dad earlier that day not to bring any money. But he brought a couple hundred dollars so we ended in a sleazy hotel and we couldn't do the things that I had planned. My parents didn't care. They were just happy that I was alive and coming home.

All year I had a picture of Golden Gate Bridge on my wall because once I saw it, I knew that I was home. On my return trip I had a military hop to Hawaii and then a military hop from Hawaii to the States. I ended up on a cargo plane with no windows, so I never saw the bridge.

When we got to the base in Oakland, we were instructed to take our uniforms off and throw them in the trash can because protesters were outside and would throw stones and tomatoes. They did anyway because those coming out that door were from overseas. My friend refused to take hers off and was spit on by drivers as she hitchhiked. Also, we had no debriefing. I was lucky enough to have friends who lived there and they picked me up. I stayed with them a week or so and they helped me reintegrate before I went home.

I saw enough death and dying to last me the rest of my life. I came home in 1970 and worked in the Walter Reed Neonatal Intensive Care Unit for four months. I found a civilian job at Fort Belvoir, Virginia. I worked on the general medical/surgical unit from November until May. I got a job in a surgical position and stayed there until 1974, when I was finally able to get back into obstetrics.

I had trouble dealing with some experiences while working in the States because of my experiences in Vietnam. One of the first cases I did when I was back in the States was done on a lung case. The longer the patient is under anesthetics the harder it was for them. The doctor asked for an instrument and the circulator ran out to get it. She returned and stated that someone had not autoclaved it. He proceeded to throw a temper tantrum. He folded his arms and said, "I'm not doing anything until I have my instrument." It would take about 30 minutes to autoclave it. It was very hard because in Vietnam we did major cases with a minor instrument set. We didn't have all the fancy instruments. The doctors did amazing things with a basic instrument set. But yet this doctor couldn't deal at all without one instrument. My thought was, "Send the sucker to Vietnam." Getting back to the States we were not allowed to start IVs until we took the IV class. While in Vietnam we often had to start IVs on our knees holding a flashlight in the dark!

There are lifetime consequences of war. The type of wounds incurred by veterans coming home will be present all their life. Statistics show that one in three returning veterans have PTSD. I don't think that there's anything important enough to go to war. America will not be great for the amount of wars that it has fought but will be great when it learns how to establish peace and teaches that to other nations. Never forget the high price of freedom, a price every veteran and their family has paid!!!

Mitchel A. McDonald

Though the actual account of Mitchel A. McDonald's experience in Vietnam is short, so much of his professional life following that experience was influenced by his experience in Vietnam. Mitchel makes observations on the status of the enlisted man at the time of Vietnam, on the experience of a young officer and on the kindness and insight of his senior officer.

In 1965 I was given the tremendous opportunity to give up my $1.75 per hour job at a car wash to go to work at a hospital as an orderly. I was about 20 years old and still partying, studying and working full-time. With the Vietnam War going on I felt that if I joined the Navy that there would be tremendous educational opportunities and it would help me figure out what I really wanted to do with my life. I didn't have a draft number because I was in college at the time.

I signed up for the Navy. The stipulation on the contract was that I would go to San Diego because they had hospital corps school there. Somehow I was able to look at my orders before I took my oath and I found out that they were going to ship me to the Great Lakes, Illinois. I talked with the chief and told him that since the Navy wasn't keeping the promise for me to go to San Diego, they probably would not keep their promise on a lot of things. I left and when I was about six blocks from the recruiting center the chief caught up to me and said, "It's been a horrible mistake but it's been corrected. We found that you were indeed signed up for San Diego and you are guaranteed. Now you're going to San Diego." I ended up in San Diego later in the summer.

I went to work in the San Diego Naval Hospital. I worked up on the SOQ (Senior Officer Quarters) wards for a while and then went down to the emergency room. While in the ER, we had one really tough night. We had a couple of gunshots come in and a couple of cardiac patients arrested. It was a hellish night but everyone lived through it and we had them all tucked in. It was about three in the morning and one of my colleagues in

128

the ER was giving me a neck rub when the chief nurse of the hospital walked through. She was tremendously impressed with the fact that a female corpsman was giving a guy a neck rub in the center of the ER. The next morning we both had to show up in her office and we were chewed out. We were in trouble and we couldn't work together so she was shipped off to another department in the hospital. There were still things pending up in the air because it was frowned upon from a disciplinary standpoint. Within two weeks I was in Vietnam and she was in Italy.

During my time in San Diego I went up to Long Beach for a long weekend to visit old friends from Wisconsin. While we were gone, a set of orders came in with my name on them. It was unheard of then for the enlisted to receive named orders. They were usually blanket orders for example, "send twelve people." Once they received the name orders they couldn't find me and so they sent the notice to my sister's address even though she had moved three or four times. By the time I returned, the rest of the group had been on 15-minute notice for three days. Ultimately the decision was that if I got on the plane, I was going to an exotic place in the east, my former and present master chief would make sure that 19 charges made against me would be dropped. They were dropped and I ended up in Da Nang in August 1967 until late August 1968. My back rub in the ER seemed to have gotten attention beyond my wildest expectations.

The first person to meet us at the hospital was the executive officer (XO) from the hospital and corps school. He said to me, "You're exactly what I wanted. I hand chose you." Again we were blessed children. I spent three months working on the medicine wards. Then they needed some help in the shock trauma research unit. The surgeons in the unit were studying the effectiveness of resuscitative agents. We were able to develop some classic research that was the basis for many resuscitative measures that stood for over 20 years. We would resuscitate patients, most of whom were triple amputees or severely hypotensive with blood volume expanders. As a result we had good research data on each patient. Some of the agents were really saving lives.

One of the patients had both legs blown off at the hip. He only had one kidney left. It had kind of an egg shell fracture. One of the OR techs spent a little over an hour working on putting it back together. We then put the kidney back into the patient and hooked it up and it worked. We had to keep track of these patients that lived through this whole process. It was about four months later that the patient left us and after a series of setbacks he was sent back to Japan or the Philippines and ultimately sent back to the States.

The hospital had some of the only air conditioning available, which could be affected by the attacks on the hospital. But we had one area that never lost its air conditioning because it was a self-contained unit. One day I was sitting there typing and I was crying my eyes out. There was just so much work to be done. I was a bit discouraged. Many patients didn't survive because of the severity of the injuries and a lot of the resuscitative measures were still in their infancy. I dropped the letters in the mail and picked up the new mail that had just arrived that day. There was a picture of a guy skiing in Colorado, one of our previous patients. That was when I really had a true faith experience that miracles were happening every single day.

At the same time we had a patient who had been star baseball pitcher. He had been engaged to a beautiful beauty contest contestant. He had an ankle fracture which led to some problems and he figured that he would never be the same. Eventually he was infected, septic and ended up dying. It was a stark contrast between the patient with the ankle fracture, which was not too bad on the relative scale, compared to the patient with both legs blown off. Part of the significance of the ankle fracture patient was that he felt that he could no longer be a pitcher. When he was no longer a winner for his team and they didn't need him anymore, he became cannon fodder for the draft. He went to Vietnam less than a year later. He went from world class baseball hero to Joe Schmuck and ended up dying. Essentially he felt his life was over and that he could no longer be the man for his beauty. That experience really fostered a lot of spirituality and growth for me.

Upon getting ready to leave Vietnam the doctors tried to get me to go to Bethesda with them. They were heading up a neophyte transplant team back at Bethesda working on transplantation of kidneys. It was in its early days of research in that area. I declined the opportunity. I got orders to go to the Naval Air Station in Albany, GA in September 1968. After settling there for a couple of weeks I was promoted from a third to a second class petty officer.

I was discharged out of the Navy in February 1970 as an enlisted person. I was working at Johns Hopkins Hospital and enrolled in their RN training program. While I was working, I went to school full-time and they gave me extra pennies along the way. I was enrolled as a student at the University of Maryland but was in the process of transferring over to Hopkins because they were going to pick up the bill.

The doctors were teaching some of us how to do surgery in the hyperbaric chambers. I was gullible enough to think that it was such a cool job. Then one night as I was taking the bus home I started to get some of the nitrous reaction from being in the chamber for too long. I had to go back to the chamber to decompress. While I was sitting in there for another four and a half hours decompressing, it finally dawned on me the reason why they had someone like me in here instead of them was because it was a dangerous environment. The reality hit me square between the eyes and I didn't want to do it anymore. By that time the other guys were willing to do it and I didn't have to.

One day we had a businessman who had been hit by a drunk driver, medevaced out and admitted into the hospital. We resuscitated him for 12 hours. After about three days the hospital administrator called his wife and three kids and he was going to meet them at the bedside. The patient (husband and father) was on a ventilator and was going to be on it for about another three weeks. The hospital administrator had just found out there was no insurance. The hospital administrator wanted his money. I remember vividly the wife saying, "Where am I supposed to get one hundred thousand dollars?" That was a lot of money back then. The hospital administrator looked at her coldly and said, "You have a beautiful home that is nearly paid for and you have three kids in college, and you're not working and neither are they and we need our money." That day I decided that the military health-care system, where privates get the same care as admirals and generals and everybody in between, had some merit to it.

I went back down to talk to my recruiter while the war was still going on. I was still going to school full-time and working on more credits. The Navy Nurse Corps Candidate Program picked me up. I was able to go to school for a couple of years drawing E5 over 6 pay by that time. My wife and I were both working full-time so life was good. We did not have any kids.

I graduated from University of Maryland in 1973 and afterward went down to Portsmouth, VA. I was supposed to go to OIS (Officer Indoctrination School) in late June or July but something was screwed up so it was pushed back to August. We had already bought a house and we had invested all of our savings in this house because I thought that I was going to be the shining new ensign making lots of money. Well it didn't happen until the end of September. Back then commission officers couldn't have a part-time job so I couldn't get a job. We used up all of our money. We were literally collecting pop bottles for gas and for food. I was an ensign. I couldn't work until I was through with OIS.

My Vietnam experience had an impact on my experience as a Naval officer. Tet, 1968, was tough time for everyone in Vietnam. The hospital in Da Nang frequently received mass casualties, 20 to 30 of them at a time, 24 hours a day. One thing that created consternation was when the media would report that the US forces had overwhelmingly defeated everybody that week and that there had only been 200 casualties through the entire I Corps area. When we counted them up, sometimes more than that had come just into our facility. So there was a little bit of contrast between what was reported in the media and the real hard facts. Even though the hospital could hold only 250 patients there was one 24-hour period that we admitted more than 250 patients.

One night during Tet, I must have fallen asleep. We were working 20 to 30 hours straight for weeks on end. I woke up and there was the chief nurse, Mary Cannon, taking care of my patients for me. She went about her business and asked me if I got a nice little snooze and I responded "Yes." She then moved on to covering the rest of the house and I reassumed my duty. Several years later, after OIS, when I checked in at Portsmouth, she was the chief nurse there! I thought that I had it made and was a special blessed child. I checked in at Portsmouth and promptly sat down at the chief nurse's office. I came to the realization that maybe a life as a baby ensign was going to be a little bit different when she asked me why I sat down without being offered a seat. I expected that I would be assigned to ICU because of my past experiences. When she told me that I was going to pediatrics and not ICU, it was heartbreaking. She then told me that if she had anything to do with it, I would never work in another ICU again. She felt I had seen more than my share of trauma and that I didn't need any more of it. So I went up to pediatrics and after about a year or two she retired and went down to South Carolina to play golf for the rest of her life. She was wonderful, compassionate, insightful and tough as nails. I now realize her brilliance too, at her compassion for and protection of me.

I spent a couple of years at Portsmouth working a variety of areas. I helped set up a nurse orientation and hospital corpsmen orientation program which was brand new back then. I then went to Hospital Corps School and was an instructor for a few years. When I was getting ready to finish up my tour, my wife ended up getting pregnant. By that time we had a couple of pregnancies, some of which didn't turn out real well. We had two little girls by then. She was due to deliver at the same time that I was supposed to go to Japan. Fortunately I was able to stick around for the baby to be born. It was going to be an obligation of a minimum of one year and a maximum of eighteen months unaccompanied. I wanted to do them, and the family was ready for that.

We ended up having an infant son with osteogenesis imperfecta and 89 fractures at birth because of the disease. Some of the fractures started to heal and other new fractures developed. He wasn't supposed to be born or live an hour or even six hours. Meanwhile he was transferred from the Great Lakes to Chicago. When we arrived at the Chicago hospital, we were told that babies born with the disease usually never survive after birth. But our son survived and it was all in God's hands. Ultimately he lived to three weeks old and we were getting ready to take him home the next day. The previous night, around 10 P.M. or 11 P.M., when we returned home, we received a phone call from the hospital. After we had left the hospital, he had gotten sick and by the time we got back to the hospital he had died. The beauty of it was that people from all over the world came together to support us in our moment of need. We were able to really see what the "Navy family" really meant. It was a very spiritual experience. It was tough for everyone, but we received a tremendous response from people we had met years before and others coming out of the woodwork, so to speak. It was a very heartwarming and endearing experience.

In preparation for the trip to Japan our middle daughter was in kindergarten and there she told all her buddies that her father was going to Japan and was going to send her kimonos and Japanese dolls. When fall arrived and everyone in the 1st grade did their show and tell, she never showed up with any of the kimonos or Japanese dolls, so her real close buddies called her a liar. My orders to Japan had been cancelled because the Navy didn't want to send me halfway around the world because of the baby's death. However, after Kellie's experience of being called a liar, my wife and I decided it was time to move on with life. A week later I ended up going to Iceland. My family was supportive of it. (Kellie finally got her Japanese dolls after a short vacation there 25 years later).

Mitch served in Iceland. He returned to go to graduate school at Marquette University in Milwaukee, graduating in 1983 with a master's in medical/surgical nursing and a certificate as a clinical specialist. He served at Camp Lejeune, a Marine Corps Base in North Carolina, and stayed there for about four years.

He was picked up as an advisor to the surgeon general, working on getting ready for the next war, though they didn't know where or when it would occur. He had over 20 years of service in the Navy by then. He served in Portsmouth as a clinical specialist in orthopedics. He served on the USS Guam, *an amphibious assault carrier, in the Mediterranean before retiring.*

My experiences at Vietnam made me who I am today. In looking at my war experience, Mary Cannon was a tremendous leader, mentor and director during the experience in Vietnam. I arrived in Vietnam at the same time the first nurses got there. I remember patients dying of tetanus and ascaris. Their bodies were weakening due to other disease entities and they were choking because of the ascaris. I remember one night I was assigned to the "holding" tent and had six patients die on me one night. The holding tent was a triage system, depending on the wounds and the needs of all the patients and resources. Losing sick patients, even though they were "expectant," was tough. I also felt that it was a healthy experience especially since I had good faith in God. Lots of people have different mechanisms to cope. But overall as a result of decent parental upbringing, some faith experiences along the way, good friends, lots of luck and faithful family members, things have turned out pretty well.

The Navy continues to be a significant part of my life as I continue to work as a civilian in orthopedics at Portsmouth Naval Hospital. Attempts at helping people cope with life changing events continues to be challenging and rewarding. Every day I am honored to work with today's heroes like those motorcycle and trauma victims where insight and peace of days past affect the lines of military personnel and their families. My friend from high school days has now been my wife for over 36 years. Our life focuses a lot on people living on the margins of society throughout the world and family. A deep faith in God and sharing our gifts from God seems natural. We anticipate using the gifts we have to be tools for God's hands just like in the days of a young corpsman in Vietnam.

My thanks to friends, such as Ed LaVenture and Mary Cannon, who continue to be mentors on life experience 101. My parents, parents-in-laws family, especially my wife, Karen, have always been available and supportive in reminding me of God's love and care. Thanks also to Pat Rushton and the Nurses at War Project for allowing me to share and reflect on a challenging time of war and post-war insights of a young "lead steamer," hospital corpsman and nurse.

Shalom

Mary Lou Ostergren-Bruner

The next account is another very personal story of a nurse's experience on the front in Vietnam. It imparts to the reader the physical and emotional situations nurses found themselves in when serving in-country. It expresses a desire for education, nursing experience and adventure, addresses naïveté we have already seen about the war and the developing reality of the situation, and their feelings toward patients, colleagues and country.

My father instilled in me the principles of patriotism, serving our fellowmen, and doing something for your country. He taught those principles by example and so my later choices to be a nurse, join the military and service in Vietnam felt natural.

When I graduated from nurses' training in the 1966, I worked at the Minneapolis Veterans Hospital, as the need for nurses was great. During that year, I came to appreciate what these men and women did for their country. There was a special bond among the patients and respect for one another. I decided in spring 1967 to join the Army.

Vietnam was in the newspaper and on TV. I knew a war was going on, but I knew the military was all over the world. I didn't plan on Vietnam, but planned on seeing the world and having a new experience.

I took my oath of office May 1967 with my mother and sister at my side. In July my best friend's brother, a Navy corpsman, was killed in Vietnam. We spoke little of this loss then, even less later. I imagine it was not easy to see a friend leave for military training shortly after her brother's death.

I was a loner at this point. I didn't join on the "buddy system" and could not bring myself to sign on as a student nurse. In September 1967, classes at Fort Sam Houston were very large, 350 to 360 medical personnel including doctors, dietitians, dentists, and nurses, all officers. Upon my arrival, there was no room on base, so we were housed in a small hotel. Training sessions were held to learn how the military operated in such areas as etiquette and how to wear the uniform. A few days were at Camp Bullis learning to use a compass, how to use a gas mask, hold a .45 revolver, touring a mock Vietnamese village, practicing triage on the injured in a tent hospital, traching a goat and watching old films from the archives.

We kept hearing about deployment to Vietnam right out of basic training. People were upset and had been clearly misled by recruiters. If I was going next, I needed more experience. When the opportunity came up for the operating room course, I requested it, knowing in my heart it would be helpful.

I received orders for Letterman Army Hospital, San Francisco, California. Part of the training as OR nurse was to train the OR technicians, some of whom ended up in Pleiku, Vietnam. The OR class was cut short due to a growing need in Vietnam. After 30 days back in Minneapolis to say my goodbyes, I departed for Travis Air Force Base. A classmate and I boarded our plane for Vietnam; a commercial airline. We were the only females onboard besides the stewardesses. Twenty-four hours later we landed in Long Binh. The heat and smell in Long Binh was sickening. The heat was humid, like Minnesota summers, but the stench was indescribable. I smelled that again years later watching the movie *Platoon*, even though I was nowhere near Vietnam.

We were allowed to request our duty assignments since nurses were needed everywhere in Vietnam. My friend and I were split up. She said to the chief nurse, "I'm a California girl. I want to be on the water." She was sent to Chu Lai. I said, "I've never really been in the mountains, being from Minnesota, so, I'll take the mountains." I was assigned to the 71st Evacuation Hospital, Central Highlands, Pleiku.

From Long Binh to Pleiku we traveled by a C130 cargo plane. We were placed in back. Only sling seats back there and not knowing how to use them, we sat on the floor, dress uniform and all, and just held on tight. I met a married couple going to the same hospital who became good friends over the next year. This was one of those many moments I asked myself what I had gotten into.

I never saw anything like it. First day on duty, I was not prepared, even after looking at the training films they showed us in basic training. Every wound was filthy. There were guys with legs and feet missing, gaping chest and abdominal wounds, and arms barely attached. We used gallons of normal saline to rinse wounds. They were debrided or cleaned out and

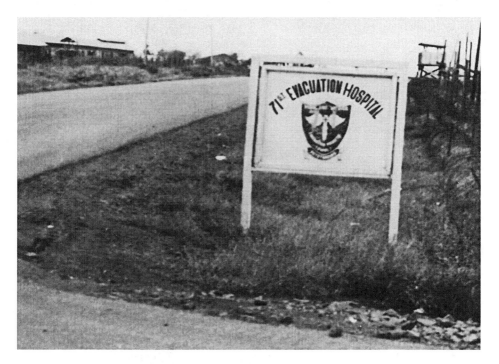

Entrance to the 71st Evacuation Hospital, Pleiku.

left unsewn. They were filled with gauze and wrapped to come back another day for more debriding. You also had gaping head wounds and facial trauma. Amputees were frequent. A lot of times it wasn't just an arm, but it was more than one limb. They were all young and they look like your kid brother. We had every type of MD and surgical specialist at the 71st and we kept them all busy. If a physician's specialty wasn't on our table in the OR, he could always assist another surgeon.

Neurosurgeries or head cases were the most difficult to take. The corpsmen, like me, worried about the outcome. I always scrubbed, so they didn't have to. I think we hated those cases because losing an arm did not mean your life was so very different, but losing who you are; not recognizing family and friends, not enjoying the life you remembered was not easy for us to think about. Life expectancy was tenuous, infection was common. One corpsman, years later, told me I always had tears in my eyes during such cases.

At first, I was checking names of the wounded and finding out where they were from. States close to Minnesota found me connecting and chitchatting. Then I stopped as the wounds intensified and the numbers increased. All of a sudden it was too personal, too hard to handle.

Upon arrival we worked eight-hour days and took call. Many a night I was awakened and called to work. Shortly after I arrived, we went to twelve-hour shifts, six days a week. Blaring sirens sounded with red alerts and rocket attacks. These would send me hitting the floor of the hooch, usually at night. As the rockets whished overhead and thudded into the ground, making the earth shake, my roommate and I took shelter together and prayed the rosary. I decided if I was going to spend nights wearing a flak vest and helmet and seeking shelter under the bed, I would rather be working. I requested night duty from 7 P.M. to 7 A.M. I was the only nurse on the shift working with six corpsmen. When busy due to a "push" with multiple casualties and running all five operating rooms, we would call in some of the day shift. I often worked twelve plus hours.

The littlest things kept us going, boosting our morale. These were things like celebrating someone's birthday with a cake baked in an electric fry pan, talking endlessly of one's plans for return to the world or the compound gossip, planning gag gifts for the staff at Christmas, decorating a tree branch for the holidays, sharing mail and "care packages," complaining about the higher-ups and the white-glove inspections and especially the food. We shared stories of R&R trips to Japan, Hong Kong, and Australia. We had Friday night steak fries and dances with live bands, which were usually lip-synching Filipinos. They were actually quite good.

We played tricks on one another like filling out paperwork for surgery for Colonel Clause and a party of eight injured as his aircraft came down Christmas '68, then calling the head nurse out of bed in the middle of the night. We could have been in reindeer poop big time, but she had a great sense of humor.

Our compound was the size of several city blocks surrounded by concertina wire, a lot of dirt and little greenery. Looking into the distance you could see the higher elevations. The Fourth Infantry Division was on Dragon Mountain and we were in the valley. We had a Special Forces Camp relatively close as well. They worked with the Montagnards, who were native to the area and were our allies.

The hospital was made up of Quonset huts forming a cross. They housed the emergency room, x-ray, lab, surgery and recovery. At the time, mid '68–'69, the hospital had seven wards and close to 600 beds. Our main

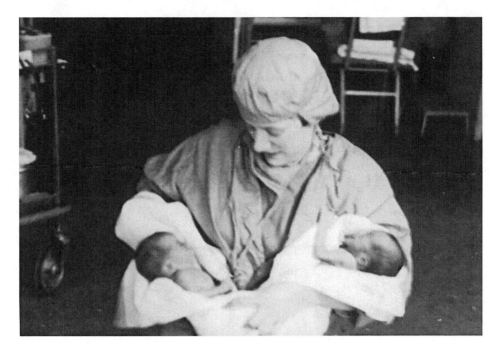

Vietnamese babies born November 1968.

duty was to stabilize and evacuate patients for more surgery and or recovery to convalescing hospitals in-country and out of country, such as to Japan. We were both a surgical hospital and a medical facility. We had enlisted barracks, an enlisted club, theater, pool, chapel, Red Cross building, hospital headquarters, recreation hall, officers' quarters, officers' club, volleyball court and a small post exchange and barbershop. A Vidal Sassoon stylist visited during this year to give the nurses haircuts.

We had guard towers, similar to a forest ranger's tower, but not as tall, overlooking the countryside. These were manned by our hospital corpsmen after a 12-hour shift. Our neighbors were engineers stationed on Radar Hill at the old 18th Surgical Hospital at the ARVN Camp. There was an Air Force base up the road a bit from the city of Pleiku. For exercise and entertainment we walked to other bases to visit post exchanges and to downtown Pleiku. Occasionally we got a ride in a jeep, a "deuce and a half" or a taxi called a Lambretta. It was a way to see the lush, green countryside, which was not as stark as our compound. Except for R&R, we were restricted many times to the compound during "high alerts."

Weather was overall mild, windy, and cooling down in the evening, making it almost pleasant. The monsoons were another story. It rained so hard it looked like night all day. We wore ponchos over the uniform to stay dry. An umbrella would have been ripped to shreds. We had deep trenches on either side of the walkways so the rain just ran off the flat ground and filled the trenches. Our hooch never flooded, but every article of paper, bedding or clothing was damp. I don't remember how long the rains lasted, days or weeks. Some of the smells I believe were due to the high humidity. Everything lingered in the air. We had metal lockers in our rooms in the hootches. To keep mildew from growing up the sides, we hung a bare electric bulb inside. As we turned in our summer dress uniform and heels for fatigues and combat boots, the stateside articles went into the locker for the next year.

This country, halfway around the world, was primitive. There were no sturdy buildings, super highways, running water or electricity in the Highlands. The Vietnamese and Montagnards lived off the land, farming and making a life now totally disrupted by war. The Pleiku Hospital was damaged by bombs and the ill and injured came to the 71st. We also visited the villages and brought medicine to them. If someone needed surgery, we brought them to our hospital with the entire family in tow. This aid was suspended during "high alert" because of enemy activity in the area and when we were busy with the wounded.

One day, one of our docs had been sent the ingredients for an Italian feast. He wanted to treat the entire OR staff. There was a community room on the officer side of the compound so everyone was assembled ready to eat when one of the company commanders appeared and sent all of the enlisted back across the line that divided us. It was okay for officer and enlisted to work alongside one another but not to share a meal. The mess hall was divided as well.

One evening at the officers' club, in walked actress and comedian Martha Raye, dressed in her Green Beret and Special Forces uniform with her photo journalist, Sean Flynn. I grew up watching black-and-white films of his father, Errol Flynn. This was a high-light. They had come to visit our patients. They did so frequently. Later, we learned Sean Flynn never returned from Vietnam, having possibly been captured or killed.

In August 1968 we received a GI with multiple injuries. We called just about every surgeon on base and hours of surgery ensued; eye, facial, neurology, orthopedics. One particular doc would not give up on this young patient. Back then you did not have the resources or time to follow everyone's outcome. Years later, this doc found our patient married with a family. He was happy even though his blindness and amputations were visible reminders of what this GI went through. He was glad to be alive. A television special and magazine article allowed the rest of us to know about this great outcome. This knowledge allowed us hope and peace in knowing it was all worth it.

One moment, meaningful beyond words, was the welcome home parade in November 1993 in Washington, D.C. We had come to dedicate the Vietnam Women's Memorial. People lined the streets and at the end stood a patient from the 71st Evacuation Hospital calling out my name. He had come to our surgery in March 1969 and had come to the parade to personally say thank you to me. Thanks are few and that's okay because I recently learned 98 percent of all wounded making it to a hospital during the Vietnam War survived.

Tears still fall freely, the days of Vietnam are not behind me, but rather they are part of me. The stories are unending, but the pages here are limited. When asked, "How did you make it?" I answer, "By the grace of God and with family support through prayers and mail and the greatest team of coworkers in all of Vietnam.

As of 2012, I am still in the Minneapolis area and married for over 40 years to the man who remains my biggest cheerleader, telling all who will listen that he is married to a veteran. We have two children and five grandchildren. We are blessed. I live by our motto in Vietnam, "Remember the good times" and pray for peace.

Ruth E. Purinton

Ruth E. Purinton landed in Vietnam in the very early days of the war, having volunteered to be one of the first 18 Navy nurses assigned to the Naval Support Activity Hospital in Da Nang in August 1967. She was essentially a pioneer in caring for troops in the war zone. She speaks of the experiences and challenges of caring for seriously wounded troops there. Ruth expresses her gratitude that the wounded were provided exceptional medical and nursing care so quickly after being wounded. She speaks of the difficulty of returning home and the support of family and friends in making the transition less stressful.

I had always wanted to be a nurse. After I graduated from high school at Pinkerton Academy in Derry, New Hampshire, in 1953, I applied to several nursing schools. I was accepted at the Peter Brent Brigham Hospital in Boston, Massachusetts. Graduating in 1956, I started at the hospital, working for Dr. Dwight Harken as a cardiovascular nurse. This was an exciting position. Dr. Harken was the pioneer in cardiac surgery and valve replacements with patients coming from all around the world to have this renowned surgeon perform their heart surgery.

After several years at the Peter Brent Brigham Hospital, I accepted a position at the Mt. Sinai Hospital in New York City in the recovery room, assisting with their open-heart surgery patients. I decided that military nursing would provide me with excellent nursing experiences, plus I would be seeing a lot of unique places.

I went to the Navy recruiter in New York, but the Navy did not need any nurses for at least nine months. I went to the Air Force recruiting office and filled in the extensive application and in several weeks, I received a telegram that I was accepted for a commission in the United States Air Force Nurse Corps.

As part of my application to the Air Force, I had requested hospitals in California, Florida and Texas. The acceptance telegram that I received stated that I would be assigned to the US Air Force Base, Sidi Slimane,

Morocco. I called the nurse recruiter immediately and stated that there must be a mistake in my orders, as I had requested California, Florida, or Texas. She said that it was not a mistake. Even though the Air Force did not usually send a person overseas for their first assignment, she felt that with my experience and maturity I could be assigned overseas for my first assignment. So, off to Morocco I went, staying almost two years. The Moroccans would not renew the lease for the base and the hospital and the base were closed. Some change from a big hospital in New York City to Sidi Slimane, a very small hospital, a B-52 base surrounded by sand.

To finish out my two-year obligation in the Air Force, I was assigned to Beale Air Force Base in California. After completing my two years of active duty, I stayed in the reserves in California and went to flight school in Montgomery, Alabama. The reserve unit I was assigned to was responsible for medevacuating patients to and from bases in Korea to Travis Air Force Base Hospital in California.

I stayed in San Francisco, trying to get my nursing degree and working part-time at a local hospital to pay the bills and keep my nursing skills current. The Navy Nurse Corps was still on my mind and I applied for and received a commission in the Navy in 1965. After officer indoctrination at Newport, Rhode Island, I was assigned to Naval Hospital, Portsmouth, which was a large teaching hospital, where I had the opportunity to update my clinical skills. I was assigned to the surgical intensive care unit (SICU) and my supervisor was LCDR Bobbi Hovis. I enjoyed working in the SICU, as that had been my area of expertise in the past.

In 1966, the Vietnam conflict was escalating and Captain C. Edwina Todd was the director of nursing at the Naval hospital at that time. She was asking for volunteer nurses to go to the US Naval Support Activity Hospital in Da Nang, Vietnam. I was seriously considering volunteering, as I thought that my extensive critical care skills and my flight nurse experiences would be beneficial in taking care of the casualties. I first discussed my decision to volunteer with LCDR Hovis, as she had been in Saigon during the conflicts there. She encouraged me to volunteer. I talked with Captain Todd. She had served in World War II and had been a prisoner of war in the Philippines. She encouraged me to volunteer and recommended me for the assignment to Da Nang.

I was very pleased and a little apprehensive to go to Da Nang. I went to Washington, D.C., for a briefing to go to Vietnam. Eighteen Navy nurses were selected to go to Da Nang in August 1967. CDR Mary Ford

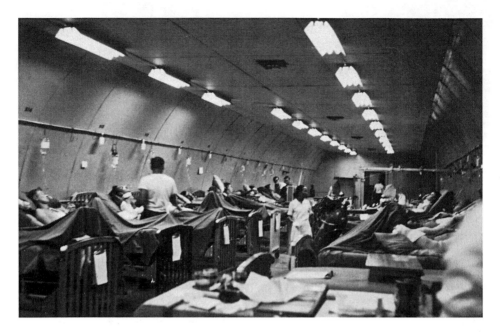

Ward in Vietnam.

Cannon was the director of nursing services and under her capable direction, the Navy nurses got the wards cleaned up and running very efficiently in a very short period of time. Casualties were coming in on a daily basis. As in past conflicts, when the first women were assigned to a medical facility, the doctors and corpsmen seemed to resent them being in the war zone. As time went on, they realized our value in helping them. We worked as a well-functioning team, which helped immensely with casualties increasing every day.

The location of the Naval Support Activity Hospital in Da Nang posed some serious problems for the patients and staff as the hospital was located in front of and across the street from the helicopter base. The base was a prime target for the Viet Cong, but because of their utilization of very primitive rocket launches, some rockets fell short and hit the hospital first.

While I was stationed at the hospital from 1967 to 1968, several parts of the hospital were hit with serious consequences. One rocket hit the urology clinic and demolished the building. Fortunately, no one was in the building at the time but the building needed to be rebuilt. Another rocket hit the surgical ward and several post-operative patients received shrapnel wounds and had to return to surgery. We tried to evacuate the patients as soon as their conditions were stable to hopefully prevent re-injuries. Still another rocket hit just in front of the intensive care unit, injuring a corpsman that was running out of ICU to obtain blood for a patient in the unit. The corpsman went to the OR to remove the shrapnel from his neck. The surgery was successful and the corpsman wished to continue his duties in Da Nang once he fully recovered.

When the hospital siren sounded, we took cover either in our quarters, covering our heads with a helmet and putting on a padded flight jacket. If we were on the wards, we would cover the patients with heavy blankets as quickly as possible and seek cover for ourselves. It took a long time to get over the sound of that siren and my response to it. Even fire trucks making that siren sound bothered me at first when I got back to the States.

In January 1968, during the Tet Offensive, the casualties kept coming in large numbers. We had to helicopter them to the hospital ships, the *Repose* and the *Sanctuary*, that were off the coast of Da Nang. There were so many casualties during the Tet Offensive that the hospital in Da Nang could not take care of all of them.

The hospital itself was under attack and the Marines managed to hold the enemy off or the hospital would have been taken, as well. Bullets were hitting all over the hospital, which meant that the enemy was very near. We were still able to treat the casualties as they were brought into the hospital from the triage area. It seemed as if the casualties would never stop coming and the offensive would never end. It did, and even though the staff was exhausted, we were grateful we were able to function so well as a team and treat so many. I am sure that many lives were saved due to the excellent rapid medical treatment in the field by the brave hospital corpsmen, the courageous helicopter pilots that quickly brought them to the hospital under fire, and the well trained and dedicated hospital staff. We worked and worked and worked, day and night. It didn't matter. All we wanted to do was save and treat as many of our troops as possible.

We did go on R&R to Bangkok, Thailand, on one trip and to Hong Kong several months later. We got our hair and nails done and had a short rest. I didn't really enjoy it that much. I was just so concerned with what was happening back in Da Nang and knowing how many people were getting killed, wounded and contracting various medical illnesses. We really couldn't have a good time because we knew all the horror that was going

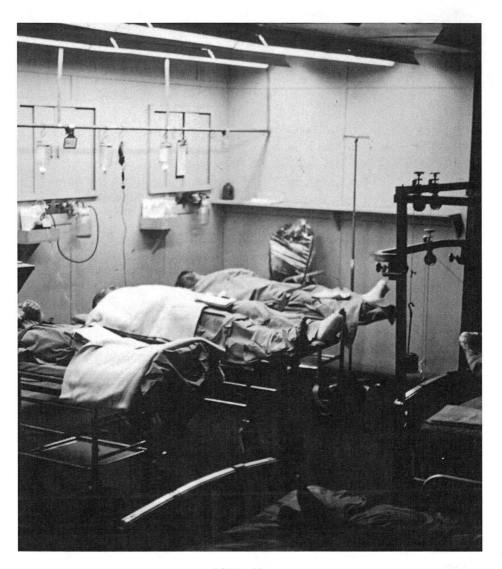

ICU in Vietnam.

on. I wanted to go back and help. I wasn't afraid at all. It was just a matter of how sad this all was. You'd see people in the dining room on vacation and having a grand time. You'd think, "Do you have any idea what's happening in Vietnam?" It was just such a contrast between coming from the devastation in Vietnam to Hong Kong where everybody was on vacation

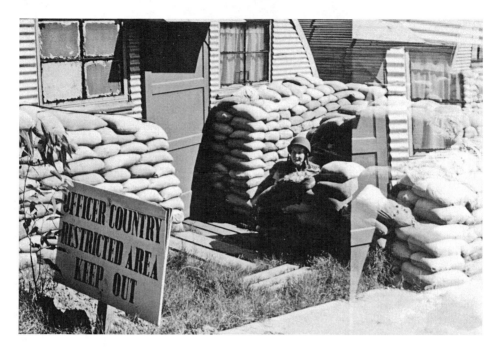

Ruth E. Purniton outside sandbagged Quonset hut.

having a great time and seemed oblivious to what was going on in the world. I think today we're all very well aware of what is going on in Iraq and Afghanistan. Vietnam wasn't as televised. You didn't have reporters with the troops. When you looked at these people outside Vietnam, you really couldn't blame them for not knowing what was happening because they had no way of knowing.

At the Naval Hospital in Da Nang, I was assigned to the surgical area. We had many medical patients with infectious diseases, malaria and trench foot from the troops being in swampy conditions. They were very sick and many of them died from malaria and other medical problems. I was astonished about the number of medical patients that die in a war zone before coming to Da Nang. I was mainly focused on the wounds that were caused by combat. We were confronted with all kinds of casualties as the North Vietnamese would put these land mines where the troops would drive over them with their tanks. The whole halftrack would be burning and you would have all these severely burned patients all at one time. Individual troops would step on the land mines and amputate their legs. After one fierce firefight with the North Vietnamese we did 21 craniotomies for troops with head wounds. The neurosurgeons took turns operating all day and all night until all 21 craniotomies were complete. We all thanked God that we were able to treat them so quickly.

The craniotomy patients were medically evacuated by the Air Force flight crews to Clarke Air Force Base, Philippines. This was a big responsibility for the flight nurses to care for that many head injuries. These flight nurses had excellent training to transport all the injured patients safely with outstanding care, saving many lives. I really admired the Air Force flight nurses. It is one thing to have patients in a hospital, but another thing to try to manage them in flight, with all the changes in hematocrits and fluids and pressures. Of course, they had a lot of corpsmen with them. But still they were responsible for the patients because there was usually no doctor. They had physicians on the radio many times, but not on site, not on the plane themselves.

The corpsmen did a magnificent job on the front lines with the Marines. They just did everything for the wounded until they could be evacuated to a medical facility. When there was a break in the fighting, the corpsmen would come to see if the patients they had treated in the field were still at the hospital in Da Nang. They were a very dedicated and totally capable group, which I admired very much.

The generals and admirals all made rounds every Sunday. They came to see all their troops. They were wonderful about that. Occasionally we would have some congressmen or senators come see what was going on with their constituents. Martha Raye came several times. She's an OR nurse and she actually assisted in the operating room. That was very interesting that she would be willing to help out in the OR in a war zone.

We did have a little exchange, but I don't remember that we bought much in it. We took a lot of personal things with us, like female personal things, because we knew they wouldn't have those things there. If we needed something, we all would write home to our families. I remember sending home for a girdle and my sister sent me a girdle. She wrote back saying, "You're in a war zone and you still need a girdle?" Even in Vietnam we had to fit into the uniform.

Commander Mary Cannon was the chief nurse and she wanted to keep things sort of normal for us. Birthdays were coming up and so she insisted that we all have a birthday party. I was the chairman of the birthday party committee. I asked two of the nurses what kind of a cake they would like for their birthday. They wanted a small, two-layer chocolate cake. I went over to the cook and said, "We need a small, two-layer chocolate cake saying, 'Happy Birthday' on it. I'm going to be on duty. One of the nurses will come pick it up on her way off, around seven at night and take it over to the nurses' quarters for the party."

The nurse who agreed to pick up the cake came over and she said, "I'm coming to pick up the cake for the nurse corps birthdays." The cooks go in the freezer and they bring out this huge cake. I mean huge. It took two cooks and the nurse to bring it over to the nurses' quarters. While I'm on duty I'm seeing cake flying all over this hospital. I'm thinking, "My gosh, where did all this cake come from?" I got a note from Mary Cannon saying,

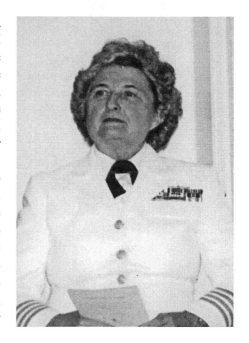

Ruth E. Purinton at retirement.

"Please see me immediately after you get off duty." I thought, "My gosh. What did I do?" She said, "Would you tell me what kind of a cake you ordered?" I said, "Yes, a small, two-layer chocolate cake saying, 'Happy Birthday.'" She said, "Did you know it took two cooks and the nurse to bring that cake over and it fed a thousand men. It weighed 48 pounds!" The cooks only had cake pans to fit a thousand men. Not only that, but the cooks were spending all their day frosting that cake. When they took it out, the frosting melted all over it. It was very hot in Vietnam. She said, "If you think that's funny, I'm going to take you off the cake committee."

I left Da Nang in 1967 realizing that our job had not been completed. There were still many troops being wounded and the conflict was still ongoing. However, when I left I did believe that our patients received the best medical care possible under such horrific circumstances. I will always remember the patients waking up and looking at us in our white uniform and asking us if we were angels. I assured them we were not angels, but that we were blessed to be there to take care of them and to get them back home to their families as soon as they were able to travel.

On the way back from Da Nang, I stopped to see Edwina Todd, retired in California, to share some of my Da Nang experiences. She was very supportive of the Navy's medical department effort to have the best medical and nursing care in her war experiences and in the current conflict in Vietnam. She was an outstanding role model for me and all the nurses that served with her.

When I came home, I just remember being awfully tired. I was assigned to Naval Hospital Chelsea, Massachusetts, which was only an hour's drive from my home in Chester, New Hampshire. I was so pleased to be near home after being so far away under such stressful circumstances. My family was very supportive of me when I returned home and assisted me in coping with the realities of war and to getting back to a sort of "normal" life.

There were several other Navy nurses that had been in Da Nang with me at Naval Hospital, Chelsea, but we rarely talked about our time in Vietnam unless it was something that was funny, like me carrying grass seed to a war zone with "Keep off Grass" signs. Today, it is difficult to watch on TV again the many young people that are being killed and wounded in Iraq or Afghanistan and my heart goes out to their loved ones as they experience the horrors of war. Until you have been there, there really isn't any way to explain how devastating war is. One can only pray that somehow the benefits of such decisions can possibly out weigh the human costs. I am glad that I volunteered to go to Da Nang to provide nursing care to the troops. If I were a little younger, I would definitely volunteer again for this present conflict.

Maria V. Rossi

Maria V. Rossi's story demonstrates the diversity of experience of military nurses. It demonstrates how their experiences build upon each other, producing continually developing clinical and leadership skills.

I went to nursing school in St. Joseph's Hospital School of Nursing in Hancock, Michigan, in the Upper Peninsula in 1963. I was kind of searching, so I took a year off after my junior year, and went to work for a year. I worked as a nursing assistant in my hometown hospital. It convinced me that nursing was where I wanted to be, so I went back to school. I graduated in 1967.

The Vietnam War was going on, but I didn't even think about it at the time. I went home to Iron Mountain, Michigan, and got my first job at Dickinson County Memorial Hospital, working on the surgical ward. After about 15 months I went to Green Bay, Wisconsin, and worked on a psychiatric ward at St. Vincent's Hospital. It was really interesting and I learned a lot. I started getting itchy feet and I wanted something different. I remembered the recruiter talking to us at school. After talking to the recruiter in Green Bay, I decided to join the Navy Nurse Corps.

They sent me to Newport in November 1969. At that point, the WOS (Officer Indoctrination School) was only four weeks. It was not just strictly nurses, but nurses and physical therapists. The class I was in was the last one for the year. There were only forty of us. We only learned to march once a week in the gym because there was snow all over, and they didn't make us march from class to class. I graduated from there after four weeks, first in my class. I don't think it made much of a difference in promotions. They pretty much stuck to the years and performance. Initially it was like 12 months, so after 12 months I was promoted to lieutenant junior grade. Then it was two years to lieutenant.

My first duty was at Jacksonville, Florida. There were three people from my graduation class that went to Jacksonville. We all lived in the

BOQ for the first six months. I worked on the orthopedic ward. We worked nights and evenings on three wards and we had 150 patients. They were not all as ill as they are today. You only had maybe 30 to 50 sick patients, and only three or four that required a lot of care. Then they transferred me to the surgical ICU and I worked in the surgical ICU until I left. They had a need and I could just work there. In about August 1970, Captain Duerk came to Jacksonville to visit. She was director of the Navy Nurse Corps then. My charge nurse told me I needed to go and meet her. I didn't want to, but she said, "You need to go and meet her. If you don't make an appointment, I'll make one for you." So I went down and talked to her, and she put you at ease really easily. She asked what my future plans were, and I told her I'd like to go overseas to Guam or Japan. She said that was interesting, and she talked to me a little bit and we ended our conversation and I left. Six weeks later I had orders to Guam. I told her if I went anytime soon that I couldn't leave until Christmas. It was important to me to be home at Christmas because my brother had died that June and I wanted to be home with my mother. They changed my orders and I got to go home for Christmas. I got to Guam on the first of January 1970.

I flew to Guam. I had to go to Travis and they had these huge flights that stopped on the way and dropped people off. Those flights were totally packed MAC flights. They took the families or unaccompanied active duty personnel. It took about 15 hours to fly over there with one stop in Hawaii. We got into Guam and were met at the airport. It was a holiday, being the first of January. The nurses were celebrating nurses around the world.

I worked orthopedics and general surgery ward, and every once in a while, I got pulled in the nursery if they needed help. I was introduced to the medevac watch. It was 1971 and we were down to getting maybe three medevacs a week coming in from Vietnam. We could get as low as 20 but as high as 70 to 75 patients coming in. At that point, the hospital was about 200 beds, but it had a potential of more because they had sunporches that had bunk beds on them. During the height of the '67/'68 Tet offenses, they had a branch hospital down on Asan, which is down the hill closer to the water. When I got there, it was closed and being used as a BOQ. We only used the sunporch beds for overflow for the people that weren't very ill, or had minor injuries. We had dependents, orthopedic, surgical, and medical wards, an ICU and an OB area.

The medevac watch system was kind of interesting. The A.M. and P.M. shifts assisted each other in getting the medevacs settled and getting those who had to work the next shift off as soon as possible so they could come back on their scheduled shift. It would take three to four hours to get everyone settled, bathed, fed and pre-op prepped if they were going into surgery the next morning. We hardly ever had medevacs back to back. There was usually a day in between. I don't know how many nurses we had. We had the watch a couple of times a week, but we only had medevacs three times a week. We didn't always know they were coming in. Sometimes we only got six hours' notice. If someone was really severely ill, they would go to Anderson Air Force Base, and be picked up in a bus or by ambulance. Anderson is on Guam, too. The island of Guam is really small—15 miles long and four to eight miles across. They have little towns there and Agana is the capital. The hospital is on the cliffs overlooking Agana and the Philippine Sea. Anderson AFB is on the northern end of the island. The hospital is about mid-island. Depending on how bad they were, they would send a doctor in the ambulance. Otherwise usually the doctors didn't go to the airfield.

I stayed in Guam for 19 months. I got there January 1, '71 and left in July of '72. It was supposed to be 18 months and I was supposed to leave in June, but BUPERS ran out of money for transfers so I couldn't get home until July. I missed my brother's wedding.

A couple of interesting things happened while I was on Guam. President Nixon stopped overnight when he was going to China for his first meeting. They have a VIP suite that was military owned, and he stayed there. They had helicopters flying all over the place when he came in. They flew his bulletproof limousine on a C–5 and dropped it off so it would be available for him on arrival and departure. The other interesting thing was a Japanese soldier was captured. He had been there since World War II. They caught him stealing shrimp from a trap and they caught him and determined that he was a soldier hiding there all those years. They sent him back to Japan. I think he knew the war was over. He had been living there all those years in caves on the island.

We had a typhoon while I was there. For typhoons all of the nurses went in the hospital and stayed until it was over. All the women seven months pregnant or more would come and stay at the hospital. We would put tape in the windows to keep them from breaking and scattering glass everywhere. Women go into labor earlier in typhoon weather because of changes in air pressure. I happened to work the night of the typhoon. It was howling. An area with mattresses on the floor in offices was set up where we could sleep in case we needed to work. There wasn't much damage, so we were pretty lucky.

From Guam I went to Great Lakes Hospital. At that point I wasn't sure I was going to stay in the Navy so I wanted to take orders in a place that was close to home. When I got there, I worked again on the orthopedic ward and I worked between orthopedics and general surgery. I made lieutenant. Once you're a lieutenant you usually get your own ward, and I became charge nurse of an orthopedic ward. That was the way it was in the States. Overseas sometimes they would have somebody junior be a charge nurse, but mostly it was when you were a lieutenant. While I was still a lieutenant junior grade, I got pulled into the nursery periodically when they had a lot of bad babies, but mostly I just worked surgical areas.

At this point in my career, I decided that I liked the Navy a lot and I was going to stay in, so I did my application for regular Navy. It wasn't a very long process. It was just a formality to put my paperwork in. Back then they would ask people to go regular, or be recommended from someone higher. Sometimes people decided they wanted to go regular and they had to put their paper work in and have to be chosen, but I just had to put my paperwork in.

When the POWs came back in 1974, the sick officers' quarters (SOQ) was set up for their admission. Staff was chosen to work there. We had special classes about the dos and don'ts of taking care of them. You had to have a special badge to enter the SOQ, so they were pretty well protected. It was on the top floor, and all the exits guarded so nobody could get up there that didn't belong there. We had about fourteen POWs that went through the hospital. When they first got there, they had debriefing and then all the medical workups. If a spouse was visiting a husband and they had a "Do Not Disturb" sign on the door, no matter who called or what was happening, no one could go in, even if the United States president called. None of them stayed very long, maybe a week or ten days. Some of the guys came back to the hospital after being discharged. We had one guy that had breast cancer when he came back. He had known the lump was there for six months. He got treated for that, but he didn't last very long. I think he died within two years from his cancer because it had been there for so long.

Maria received orders to Bremerton Naval Hospital. While at that duty station she went on to get her bachelor's degree from Seattle University in 1981. She then served at Camp Pendleton, Oakland Naval Hospital and on the USNS

Mercy *during its maiden voyage on a humanitarian mission to the Philippines. She talks of that important mission.*

We had a really good group of people and all the services were there— Army, Navy, Air Force, and public health. We worked well together. The charge nurses were assigned from the Navy and then the shore facilities.

There were some preparations required for the Mercy's Philippine mission. First, a bunch of us got qualified with a 45. We also went to firefighting school. On Treasure Island they had this firefighting school and you would go there and they would show you everything—how to check the doors and how to use the hoses. We actually went into buildings that were on fire and put them out. We used the OBAs, the breathing apparatus. From Oakland almost every person that went on this ship went to this firefighting school.

The other thing that was interesting was that when we went on this cruise we had our own security. Because we are a hospital ship, we weren't armed, so we had eight Navy SEALS that roamed the decks 24/7 taking turns while we were in port. I don't think anybody really knew about them. We believed they were armed, but no one could ever say because they always had a back pack with them. They had jump suits on. They were big one-piece, big-zipper jumpers and they had those on the whole time and they walked around in twos while we were in port. They were kind of like our protection. There was a ward on one of the lower decks that wasn't used and that was where they stayed. They locked it up with a chain when they weren't in there, but they were there and that was pretty nice.

We had ten days in each city that we were at in the Philippines. Half the days, one group would go ashore. Then you would switch, and the other half would go ashore, so the nursing service was divided. In those ten days, in every one of those ports, we got one day off, one day that we could go on shore and do whatever. That worked pretty well. It was interesting. I really enjoyed that a lot.

I rode the ship home as opposed to leaving the ship at the end of the Philippine mission. We went to Papua, New Guinea and Fiji. When we were coming back, the captain of the vessel asked permission if we could go 90 miles out of our way to cross the equator at the International Dateline. We had our "Shellback Initiation," and because we crossed the International Date Line at the equator, we are all "Golden Shellbacks." That was kind of interesting because you have all these Air Force and Army people who are now Golden Shellbacks.

When we came into Hawaii, we manned the rails and rendered honor to the *Arizona*. We stayed in Hawaii for three days. The ship was divided up into three groups so everyone had to stay aboard one day and then the other two days you got off. Then we took off and came back to the States. We sailed into Oakland and there was a big celebration when we went under the Golden Gate Bridge. People threw flowers. All the firefighting ships had their hoses running, and the fire ships had the red, white, and blue water. Upon return we were granted leave. When I went back to work, I became the nursing service manpower advisor.

Maria followed her Oakland mission with service in Iceland as the director of nursing service at the Navy clinic in Reykjavik, Iceland. She returned to Naval Hospital Bremerton, Washington, and subsequently retired from that duty station.

Mary Ellen Warne

Mary Ellen Warne's story is one of being in a naval facility stateside during wartime. She was able to care for many different types of patients, including amputees and POWs, both less common experiences in any setting. She tells a wonderful love story, her own, and of knowing that family is the highest priority in her life.

My mother had been a nurse with the Veterans Administration and my aunt had been an Army nurse. My mother used to tell us stories from World War II. She was sent over on the *Queen Elizabeth* in a convoy to serve in England as a nurse for wounded soldiers there. All the ships guarded the nurses who were in the center of the convoy. It was her wartime stories that initially sparked my interest in military nursing.

I graduated from high school in 1965 in Grayslake, Illinois. I decided to go into nursing because of my family history and my work with nursing clubs in high school. I wanted a four-year degree. However, I came from a large farming family of six children and I was the eldest. It would have been a financial burden to attend a four-year college. I made the decision to attend St. Therese School of Nursing to get my three-year diploma as my mother and aunt had done.

While in school I lived in the dorm and worked on weekends as a nurse's aide. I remember back at nursing school sitting in the lounge and watching the war stories about Vietnam on the news at night. The first contact I had with the Navy was piling in a car on a Friday and Saturday evening to go dancing at the enlisted or officers' clubs in Great Lakes; often, 20 or 30 of us went.

I graduated from nursing in 1968 at age 20. After graduation I decided to get a year's nursing experience. I stayed at the school and worked on the surgical unit. After a year I decided I wanted to do something that was exciting, where I could travel. I looked into the airlines and decided against it. I decided to look into the services and talked to all three recruiters. The

157

Navy didn't send a recruiter. Two nurses from Naval Hospital Great Lakes on active duty contacted me and invited me into their home to answer all my questions. It was the most memorable experience. These two young nurses loved what they were doing. The visit sold me on the Navy. I would be a direct appointee because the service had not paid for my education, and we had been out a year. They said I could have one of three picks of any naval station. Hickam air base in Hawaii was a very tempting choice for the Air Force. We ruled the Army out right away because we didn't like the uniforms. There is something about a Navy uniform that just looks sharp. There is something even better about a Marine Corps uniform. When we heard the Navy took care of the Marines, that was the clincher to our decision. The Navy had nice big stations along the coast. We picked San Diego, Oakland, and Pensacola.

I was due to report to Rhode Island in July 1969. My roommate and I got into my new car and drove from Grayslake, Illinois, up to Newport, Rhode Island, on my first big trip away from home. I remember going into Newport because it was the first time I had seen the ocean. There were big ships, and cobblestone streets, everything was military related. Our four weeks at Newport went by very fast. The main things we all learned were to salute, properly wear a uniform, and make a bed. We learned to stand a basic inspection and the marching was pretty much substandard. We had one weekend off from Navy indoctrination, so we went spent it in Boston.

After training finished in Newport, we were given orders to report to Oakland Naval Hospital in California. The hospital was impressive because it was a brand new hospital sitting on a hill that had previously been a golf course. The hospital had a circular driveway that led to the entrance. There was an inconsistency which has forever been engraved in my mind. It would become a reminder to me of the reality I would experience over the next few years. The sight of this beautiful hospital setting was interrupted by the vision of a young officer in a wheelchair with bilateral hip disarticulations, holding his two children being pushed up the hill by his wife. Oakland was the main amputee center and neurologic-prosthetic research center for the West Coast. There were always wagon trains of young amputees wheeling around from surrounding buildings to the main hospital, going to physical therapy, and the prosthetic lab.

The first year we rotated a month at a time and were oriented to all the different units. After that we could voice our preferred specialty. I had worked a year on a surgical unit after graduation and was grateful to be able to stay in that area. The hospital offered a mixture of general surgery, vascular, urology and plastic surgery. I secured a position as charge nurse. I rotated on evenings, covering three units with about 90 patients total. Fifty to 20 patients, on average, had surgery each day.

We would get patients in from Vietnam through Travis Air Force Base every Thursday which brought in men and women from the hospitals overseas. Patients were transferred to Oak Knoll Naval Hospital in Oakland by ambulance or helicopter. We were provided a list by early afternoon detailing how many patients we were going to receive. Upon arrival, they would be sent to the ER for triage, then on to different units. On the surgical ward we admitted an average of 3 to 4 patients every Thursday. It was always a time-consuming process because each patient was evaluated by teams of physicians and was given routine testing, such as malaria treatment, parasite testing and psychological evaluations.

There were a few patients that left me with lasting memories. There was one young Marine who was the center of many stories and tales that were circulated among his fellow Marine patients. He had suffered catastrophic wounds during a firefight in Vietnam. He had lower and upper limb amputations and most of his face had been destroyed. Supposedly, not finding any signs of life, he was placed in a body bag at the front. Eventually they figured out that he was still alive. He went through at least ten surgeries that I remember at our hospital. Prior to his arrival to us he had multiple major surgeries at Da Nang. Our hospital admitted him to the plastic surgery unit where he got a nose, an eye, and had jaw and neck surgery. His face regained some normalcy to those of us who were used to seeing him, but not to the general population.

We had a lot of amputees admitted to the plastics unit because their stumps didn't have enough tissue left on them to sustain prostheses. One of the popular procedures during that time was a "pedicle graft." A flap of skin would be taken from a patient's abdomen and sewn to their arm. When the flap established circulation from the arm, it would be severed from the arm. The last step would be to attach and cast the patient's arm flap to their stump. Often, after a lot of time, procedures, and discomfort from being confined to uncomfortable positions, the flap would die.

I remember all the amputees we got. They lived in the outside barracks, waiting to be medically discharged, while still receiving treatment in our hospital. I used to hear stories about the amputee Marines, and how they used to take care of one another. They kept their spirits up and always did so well in the hospital, but had problems when they were on the outside. Staff members and comrades in the hospital never made them feel uncomfortable because they were different. It was a protective environment that helped them feel secure. When they left for weekend leaves, you would hear stories of children in shopping centers pointing out their disfigurements, setting in reality for the soldiers who would soon have to leave and live in the real world. I remember one guy telling me that the hardest part for him was going to a shopping mall and walking by a mother and her children. The kids were so innocent and would ask, "Mommy, why doesn't he have legs?" or "What's wrong with him?"

Besides amputee surgeries we saw a lot of circumcisions, and then a lot of pilonidal cysts. It seemed we always had a steady stream of corpsmen packing pilonidal cysts every day. We did a lot of TURs, and a lot of urology surgery.

The cure rate for young men with testicular cancer was almost nonexistent in the 1960s. I remember a young man off a ship who was diagnosed with testicular cancer. They had discovered it after he came back. Today they can treat it, but back then there was no treatment. I do remember him being on the unit for a long time and watching his condition deteriorate. He had a girlfriend. The day before he died he wanted to leave something for his fiancée. He was married by the hospital chaplain in his room, still awake and conscious, but the next day died with all the staff, family and his new wife at his side. He was able to leave her with military benefits and life insurance.

After I had been there for six months, I had an appendicitis attack. Working on the surgical unit, and being a young new ensign, I had top care with the chief of surgery as my surgeon. Unfortunately, even though I had the best, they let me sit for two days until my appendix became gangrenous. After surgery, I was quite ill and actually ended up with pelvic abscesses. Over the next two years I had three additional surgeries related to bowel obstructions and I signed three times for possible hysterectomies. The chief of GYN was also involved in my care. He later retired to become the head doctor at the University of Arizona Medical School in Tuscon, Arizona. Because of innovative treatments at the time, I was able to have six pregnancies.

I met my husband at the hospital; he was one of my patients. After I had my appendicitis attack and was doing my walking, I encountered two young Marine patients staring at me. My husband-to-be then waved at me, not realizing I was a new nurse. I gave him a dirty look. There was a strict fraternization policy and "problem nurses" were always given orders out to less popular duty stations. When I eventually recovered and returned to work, my husband, a patient on the plastics ward, was waiting to be boarded out of the Marine Corps. Since he lived locally, we established a relationship over the next three years after he was released to become a civilian. We eventually married on August 26, 1972.

My husband was a patient at Oakland and remembers when he had sutures in his neck. This doctor had tied these with those little round things they use for fishing. He had those all in his neck. It was a new way of doing suturing to probably cut down on scarring. I have never seen that done anywhere else. My husband was over on the plastics unit after I came back to work. He was at Oakland to be boarded out the Marine Corps because of his injuries.

My husband's story is miraculous. He was in an area which I think isn't too far from Da Nang. His unit was camping through the night in a small village and planning to head back to their main unit in the morning. During the night, they began getting mortar coming in from the village. They called in their coordinates, hoping to get air support. Friendly fire came in and hit their company of ten dead on. My husband remembered the guys in his company going down in front of him from the mortar attack. As the mortar fire approached him, he put his rifle underneath his stomach, thinking, "If I make it through this, at least I will have my rifle (to take his own life)." He vaguely remembers being hit. Blood came up his throat and he passed out. Out of his ten comrades, three including him were evacuated out. Two of those didn't make it. He was the only survivor of his company. All his doctors agree he should have never lived through that night and that he is a miracle.

When my husband went down, there was a corpsman that had only been with them a week. Their previous corpsman had been killed. The corpsman came up to him and said, "Buddy, you are going to be okay. Where is your dog tag?" It was in his boot. People carried them different places, but the idea was to keep it in your boot in case your lower extremities were separated from the rest of your body, and to prevent noise. He tried to point to his boot when blood came up into his mouth. He doesn't remember anything after that. That new corpsman did a tracheotomy on him during those crucial few minutes. My husband had a severed carotid artery, jugular, a hemo-pneumothorax, lacerated liver, and multiple shrapnel wounds. My husband arrived in Da Nang with a blood pressure of 60 over 0. I bring this up because, as far as I am concerned, the people in the field and in Da Nang had to be the best of the best in difficult circumstances. They saved his life.

He spent almost a month in the intensive care unit in Da Nang. He was eventually stable and transported to our hospital. He keeps a pair of boots up in our room. He said the guy in the bed next to him in Da Nang was a double amputee. This young sergeant said to my husband, "I kept these boots for when I go home in two months. I will never wear them and they are spit polished for you to wear." My husband still has his boots and they are still in the same spit-shine condition. He was also given some insignias from an officer who never made it back to the States.

Six years later, we returned to Oakland because the neurosurgeon in Arizona where we were living thought my husband was experiencing stroke symptoms. He wanted to know who had done my husband's carotid surgery. Dr. Deaner was the vascular surgeon who originally cared for my husband in Oakland. The physician called to see if Dr. Deaner was still in Oakland. Come to find out, he was now commanding officer at Naval Hospital Oakland. Our physician conferred with him by phone and asked if he remembered my husband. Dr. Deaner remembered my husband and also remembered me. I had once been charge nurse on his thoracic unit. My husband painted a picture for Dr. Deaner of a young combat Marine. My husband was a cartoonist who used to keep his comrades entertained by drawing pictures for them. They used to tell him "We hope we don't ever get caught in cross fire with you because all you have is pencils in your pocket." Dr. Deaner told us to bypass all the red tape and come directly to Oakland and to come straight to his office. It was such an honor to be invited in by a commanding officer. After doing immediate thorough testing, he was told "You are not having a stroke. In fact, the anastomosis they did on you in Vietnam is so good we can barely tell there was an injury."

You would expect my husband to have experienced some posttraumatic stress, but fortunately he is the most well-adjusted man. He never talks about his experiences. I have to drag things out of him to find out what happened. The only time I have ever seen him down is one time when he went to a movie that portrayed Marines in a negative way. It was one of those movies that had to do with the civilian killing in Vietnam. He came out of there and didn't talk at all for two days.

162

I have so many fond memories from working at the naval hospital. We always had inspections on Fridays and we of course always tried to outdo every other unit. My husband remembers an incident when I stood up for my corpsman, and all their hard work. On Fridays, the corpsman spent many long hours polishing floors and dusting for captain's white glove inspections. We tried to keep the patients in their rooms so they wouldn't track up the shine on the floors before inspection. One day an entourage came up and started walking down the unit. I do remember saying something to them, and I remember the corpsmen looking at me aghast. I didn't think anything of it. After this group continued on through the clean floors and left the unit one of the Corpsmen said, "Miss Meyer, do you know who that was?" I said "No." They said, "That's Vita Blue." Vita Blue at that time was one of the Oakland A's top pitchers and a media phenomenon. No one would stop me from protecting all their hard work.

I was charge nurse over 80 patients on the evening shift on the surgical units. I did this until the year the prisoners of war (POWs) came back, which was about 1971. It was an honor to be able to work with the POWs and I got picked to be one of the charge nurses.

We received 26 POWs back during Operation Homecoming. They came in two groups. The hospital closed down one of the 40-bed units and put up locked doors with Marine guards standing outside for the POWs. When we were on the unit, not only were we nurses, but we were there to listen to the POWs. We had units that were supplied with champagne, with food, with anything they wanted to eat. There was nothing too much for them. They went through the first two weeks of debriefing. Military people would come and take each of the POWs into a room. They would be tape recorded for days and days. We were trying to find out if there were other POWs or MIAs.

We ran them through all the physical and psychological testing. I think it was a real transition for a lot of them because some of these men came back to children that they had never seen, and to families that had gone on to function without them. I think there were a lot of adjustments made. I remember when the first group came back they made it a point of standing at attention when the second group came back. A lot of them didn't want to meet their relatives at the airport, so their relatives were waiting for them back in their rooms. I remember one captain had his wife and five children waiting in the room when he came back. It was a momentous reunion.

Another POW that was interesting was a Marine Corps captain. He told how the POWs would collect little threads of material. With these little threads of material they fashioned a little American flag about the size of his hand. He told me when they went through Freedom Gate at the Hanoi Hilton, they raised their hands up with these little flags and the Vietnamese took them away as they boarded the plane. So when the second group came back, the first group got an American flag and they hung it from the end of the captain's bed.

I remembered that none of them wanted soup because they had lived on soup. A lot of them had scars on their wrist and ankles where they had been bound. Some of them had to have further surgery for breaks that were never allowed to heal right. They had to go back to surgery and have bones rebroken and fixed.

They were only on the ward two months. We had a total of 26 POWs. We only had a couple of men that were enlisted. The enlisted sustained probably even more punishment. This one particular guy was a sergeant and he was in solitary the whole time. There were a lot of psych problems. Oakland had a big psych unit at the time.

My last year in Oakland, I made lieutenant. I had some great nurses that taught me. One of them was Sue Ann McCumber. She was on the *Sanctuary* or the *Repose* and she had seen it all. She was an incredible person. She probably made me the nurse I am. She made me so thorough and con-scientious. She was a real stickler. If she didn't think you were doing a good job, you might as well transfer out because she would just never let up on you. I actually established a good rapport with her. When I had my wedding shower, she came. I think it was the first time I had ever seen her show up to a junior nurse's function.

After I left active duty Navy I stayed in the Naval Marine Corps Reserve unit where we drilled one weekend a month. We did a lot with the air national guard. We had a lot of really good experiences with the reserves. I was working at a hospital in Chandler, Arizona, from 1974 to 1979. I was a very busy person. I was working evenings at a hospital and doing mornings as a school nurse. I was the first school nurse for a little migrant town called Higley. Two to three nights a week I was going to school. In 1975 I had my first child. In ten years I had six pregnancies. So by 1979 I was expecting my fourth child. At that point I was trying to go to school, work two jobs, and raise three kids under five years old. In 1981 I lost my fourth child at five months and that's when I took a step back and decided I was doing too much. I had spent 12, 13 years in the Navy and I hated to give it up. I knew that I had seven more years to go but my family became the priority. My husband used to say to me, "You know, I'm never going to have to go back into the military because I'm medically retired, but what if you get called and leave me with these three little kids." As much as I hated to, I gave it up. The Navy had been the greatest experience of my life. I would have stayed in until I retired with 30 years, but I decided I had other priorities. My family was more important.

Harry A. Wesche

Harry A. Wesche, like so many military nurses, served during two conflicts, Korea and Vietnam. He describes many details of those two wars, of being an enlisted person moving to the role of officer and nurse and talks about being a male in the nursing profession.

I went into the military right after high school graduation in Salt Lake City, Utah. I was in the enlisted ranks for about ten years. At the beginning I was sent to the United States Air Force Corpsmen School at Gunter Air Force Base in Montgomery, Alabama. While stationed there only a few weeks, Rosa Parks made her famous bus ride. On my first pass off base, I was returning by bus from downtown Montgomery back to the base. As I usually did in Salt Lake, I went to the rear of the bus and took a seat. The bus went forward 10 or 15 feet and put on the brakes so hard I slid off of my chair. The driver then said, "You, white man, up here in front of the bus."

We did not hear much about what Rosa Parks did on base. A couple of weeks later I went downtown to take some pictures. Martin Luther King's chapel is right off of the main thoroughfare in Montgomery, below the state capital. I went out into the street to get a better picture of the church. A man walking by escorted me back to the sidewalk. It was not a police officer and he was white. I said told him I wanted a picture, as this was a famous chapel. The man replied, "Not in Montgomery, Alabama." He and other white men with him did not want anything to enliven, capitalize, or broaden the problem that was going on at the time. It was a little bit of an eye opener coming from the West, where we did not have the issues of segregation.

I arrived in Alabama on Labor Day weekend in September 1955. The Korean War armistice had been signed, but skirmishes on the DMZ and on sea around Korea were still happening. Many in my graduating class were assigned to Osan Air Base, South Korea. Assignments were made according to your class standing and desires. I initially received orders to Hickam Air Force Base outside Honolulu, Hawaii, as an independent duty corpsman. During the second year of that assignment, I was sent on temporary duty to a small Pacific island, Johnston Island. The next year I was assigned to Palmyra Island during the British H bomb testing. The British were based out of Christmas Island. Our contingent on Palmyra was 75 engineers, physicists and basic support. I had a radio communication with Hickam Air Force Base if it had been necessary to evacuate a patient by evacuation aircraft. Luckily, however, there were only a few injuries requiring stitches and colds to treat. There were no serious patient incidents.

When my overseas assignment time was up and I was due to rotate, there were less than 180 days left on my enlistment. The Air Force was cutting back on active duty forces and those rotating, who were not planning on re-enlisting with less than 180 days left, were allowed to separate. They would remain in the active reserve for the duration of their obligation. Those of my age group had an eight-year obligation of which I still had $4\frac{1}{2}$ years remaining.

I was released from active duty and returned to Salt Lake City and entered an Air Force reserve unit and began college. Two years later, I was informed that my contract with the Air Force had not been upheld and I was being recalled to fulfill my obligation. However, I was given the opportunity to attend advanced training for corpsmen, which was again in Gunter Air Force Base, Alabama.

I became interested in nursing as a profession and started my education at the University of Utah in the fall. While attending the University of Utah Nursing Program, the reserve pay came in handy for expenses. Six months into my junior year an Army recruiter talked me into joining the Army, which would pay for tuition and books. On completion of school and passing state boards, I would be an officer with a three-year payback commitment. In March 1963, I was discharged from the Air Force and joined the Army. I was downgraded to a PFC in the Army after having been a master sergeant in the Air Force. My pay was less, but the Army was paying for my tuition and books, so the purchase power of my income was greater. Three months before graduation I became an officer and put on the second lieutenant insignia, "the butter bar."

I graduated from nursing school in June 1965. In September I went to the Army boot camp and basic training at Fort Sam Houston in San Antonio, Texas. In January 1966, I attended the intensive care course at

Fitzsimmons Army Hospital in Denver, Colorado. It was a six-month course, and on August 1, I was sent to Korea.

The majority of the overseas transfers were sent to Vietnam, but I was sent to Korea. They wanted me to work in the intensive care unit at the 121st Hospital. If you have ever watched the movie "MASH" or have seen the TV series, you might remember that when patients would come in critical condition they would send them to the 121st. The 121st did exist and we called it "the one too many." It was the largest hospital in Korea and was located in Bupyeong, six miles from Incheon and 30 miles north of Seoul. We were all living in Quonset huts and the hospital was in a containment type of building with ICU in the center.

Besides the occasional skirmishes, our biggest medical problem was hemorrhagic fever. A doctor from the U.S. Public Health Service had just discovered the causative agent for hemorrhagic fever in Brazil. He was sent to Korea to see if he could do the same there. The disease is only found in Brazil, Russia and Korea along the DMZ (Demilitarized Zone). People who contracted the disease were sent to the 121st intensive care unit.

Hemorrhagic fever was a nursing challenge like I have never known in my life. It was treated entirely with intake and output (I&O). The way I&Os were monitored was input equaled output or the amount that was then given the next hour. It was sometimes 20 to 30 ccs out and 20 to 30 ccs in. The body fluids were so depleted that the vessels would literally opened up and everything except the heavy cells went out into the interstitial fluids. Shock was our biggest problem. We did not have kidney dialysis, so we did peritoneal dialysis. The patients' abdomens were swollen like basketballs. They would go into renal shutdown because the Loop of Henle was plugged with all kinds of cells and there were literally no fluids to flush the kidney as all the fluid went through the open part of the vessels. This cycle would go on for about a week to ten days. Afterwards, the vessels would regenerate, close and the patient would go into a heavy type of diuresis. You would actually see the long blood coils coming through the urinary down drains in the shape of the kidney vessels. It was impressive. We did not lose one patient. One day I took a patient's vital signs and prepared the IV with the amount of fluid to be given him. Everything looked good at that moment. Then I walked out of the unit to attend a meeting and had only walked a short distance down the hall when I was paged back to the ward. I ran back and the patient had dropped into shock just after I left. That is how critical the patients were. We treated 50 to 60 patients.

Hemorrhagic fever would always come in the fall and spring. During the summer and winter there weren't any cases. Hemorrhagic fever was only found in a triangle around the DMZ and not found all over Korea. It was found at the American end of the DMZ and not the Korean end. The people we were treating were American troops. All of the cases were eventually air evacuated home once they were stabilized, usually with peritoneal dialysis. They were not put on air evacuation right away because layovers and aircraft changes took a full 24 hours to fly them back to the States. On an average, it took two to three weeks to stabilize each patient. When I was teaching later, I would always bring up their experience because people would often take I&Os lightly when they are something to be taken seriously.

I was a first lieutenant with only a year's experience as a nurse. I had received very intensive training. I set up the first EKG monitoring systems in Korea in our intensive care unit. The cardiologist was amazed that we were monitoring EKGs and telemetry as nurses. The head cardiologist taught the ICU nursing staff to read the monitors. We could identify PVCs, ventricular tachycardia (v-tach) and a normal heart pattern. The head nurse, who'd come from the Walter Reed Army Hospital in Washington, D.C., asked one of the nursing staff, "What is this?" She was told it was a monitor. She then asked "Can you read it?" She asked what a PVC was and what it meant. Also ventricular tachycardia came up and the head nurse asked what it was. The nurse replied that the heart was beating faster. The head nurse replied by saying "You mean V–tach?" She said that she couldn't read an EKG and why did we even have them? Right then the cardiologist came in and said the nursing staff was the beginning of what would happen in nursing in the future.

I came home from Korea in 1967. My military records showed that I had flown air evacuation. The Army said that they wanted me to work in helicopter retrieval or the "dustoff" testing office. In the days of the Korean War we had an evacuation pattern where the corpsmen would be with the men at the fighting front and render first aid on the battle front. The injured would be evacuated back to a battalion aid station where they would be stabilized somewhat and then would be brought back to a MASH or evacuation hospital It was a stepping stone to come back home. In Korea we had an actual battlefront with specific demarcation.

In Vietnam the front was all over the place. It created for us, as medics, a necessity for a different evacuation. The "dustoff" was the bringing of the area of evacuation helicopters to the front lines and bringing the troops back to more definitive care in a hospital. When they came back by helicopter, they did not have to stop by steps. They could come directly back to a hospital situation where they could be stabilized immediately. There were times in Vietnam when we had upwards of 100 people waiting out in front of our pre-op tent and helicopters up in the sky, circling and waiting for their time to come in.

When my three years of payback to the Army for school was completed, I wanted my blue uniform back. I went back in the Air Force. The Army had been a good experience and I would not lose any rank. The Air Force detailer told me that they needed an air evacuation commander at Hill Air Force Base, Ogden, Utah, if I was interested. As a commander of the 66th Air Evacuation Reserve Flight, I worked as one of the two full-time staff members. They warned me that this unit was up for possible closer. Their past overall inspection had not been good.

We did our flying with the 945th, a flying transport unit. Air evacuation used everyone else's military planes, as we didn't have our own. We used trips to Hawaii as long distance training flights. Two operational readiness inspections were held under my command, each receiving laudatory remarks. We were honored as the most outstanding unit in air evacuation. Members of our unit, whenever there was heavy action, we were called upon to assist in bringing home the casualties. Air Evacuations were controlled out of Clark Air Force Base in the Philippines.

There were three main routes from Vietnam to the States. One went up through Japan, where the military had a branch of the famous Fort Sam Burn Center located in Yokohama. From Japan there were two routes: One went back to the Philippines; another went to the States by way of Alaska and down to the Great Lakes Naval Hospital and on to the East Coast. The second went to San Francisco by way of Hawaii. The third went back to the Philippines by way of Guam. The military found that troops recuperated faster closer to home, so if a hospital close to home was capable of handling the injury, they were transported there.

In Vietnam there were three pick-up points: Saigon, Cam Rahn Bay and Da Nang. The nurse on temporary duty from the air evacuation squadron would set up the patient placement in the aircraft (load plans). At midnight, the nurse would call the Philippines to report placement and diagnosis. The air evacuation crews would meet about 2:30 A.M. for aircraft assignments. Aircraft had arrived the previous day with cargo and had to be converted to air evacuation. After the conversion the aircraft went to one of the pickup points. The minute we touched ground in Vietnam, the loadmasters would start opening the clamshells, which were the back doors of the C–141. The doors were completely open by the time we got to our parking spot. Ambulance buses knew where we would be and were waiting for our arrival. When it was safe to drive up to the aircraft, they would load the ambulatory patients at the front of the plane and another ambulance bus would load the litter patients at the clamshell opening. Litters were placed three to four litters high, like bunk beds. Corpsmen stationed

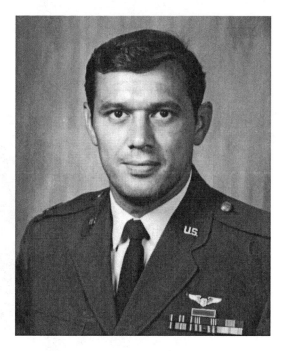

Harry A. Wesche in United States Air Force uniform.

in Vietnam would assist the aircrew corpsmen in loading by using the load plan received at midnight. Meanwhile, the nurses were receiving report on the patients. After the aircraft was loaded, it began moving down the flight line for takeoff within an hour from first landing. It was just like clockwork. The aircraft became a hospital ward at 30,000 feet. All the nursing procedures—IV's, dressing changes and TLC—that were done in a ground hospital were continued in flight. This gave the patient a complete continuance of care. This care, in addition to the knowledge that he was "going back to the world," gave the casualties of Vietnam the highest survival rate.

Upon completion of my flying assignments, I was sent to Brooks Air Force Base, San Antonio, Texas, where I attended the Air Force School of Aerospace Medicine. I completed a one-year residency in space medicine and was the first male in the space nurse program out of 20 nurses. I was sent to Edwards Air Force Base, California, to be the nurse for the first space shuttle, *Enterprise*. I was also in several other military programs, culminating in my retirement in 1983.

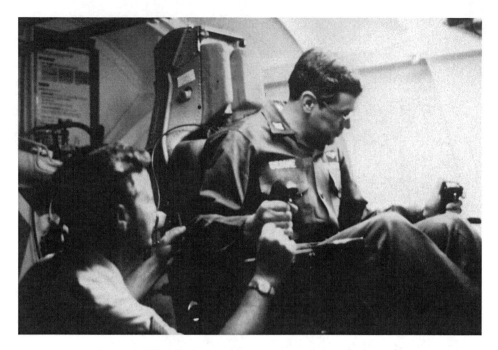

Harry A. Wesche during ejector seat training in space school.

My military experience allowed me to participate as a leader in medicine techniques and theory. Every time I was given a chance to learn something new, I jumped in with both feet. If I had it to do all over again, I wouldn't change a thing. I had professional experience, gratification and pride in a country protecting freedom and peace and a strong family's love. There isn't anything more a fellow, such as me, could want in life.

Odette P. Willis

Odette P. Willis's vast experience, as a professional and military nurse, allows her to give many details of the experience of caring for patients in many situations. She provides details that allow those who did not serve in those situations to appreciate how far nursing has developed.

I wanted to be a nurse since I was probably 10 or 11 years old. All of the guidance counselors I had in elementary and high school geared me toward math and science. I also became a candy striper for the military hospitals in Nuremberg, Germany, where I was born and raised.

My father was an Army sergeant stationed in Europe during World War II. When he got off active duty after the war, he decided to stay in Europe. He worked as a civilian in the Department of Defense for the Army and Air Force Exchange System. My mother went overseas after World War II as a computer keypunch operator. They met and married in Paris and stayed. Twenty-six years later they moved just outside of San Francisco and they have been there ever since.

We moved only once while I was growing up. I was one of two children in my family and we both started in the Nuremberg School System. I graduated from the same school 13 years later. I was both a German and an American citizen until I came back to the United States and joined the Navy. I then had to declare my citizenship and I declared the U.S. The nursing schools in Germany started you out washing floors and you worked your way up. This was the very old German school system. My father said, "No, you are going to get an education," and so I came back to the United States and went to nursing school.

I graduated from high school in 1969. I then applied to several schools in the United States, but because I was considered a foreign student, I had a difficult time getting in. I was accepted at Texas Woman's University. This is how I ended up joining the Navy. Air Force and Navy recruiters came to the campus one day during my sophomore year and talked to us about the different services. Since I was already familiar with the Army and Air Force, I thought I would take a look at the Navy. There was just something about the Navy I liked better than the Army or Air Force.

I joined the Navy in 1971 and accepted was in the Officer Candidate Program. I finished my last two years of school in this program. I graduated from college in 1973 and entered the July officer indoctrination class at Newport, Rhode Island. My parents were happy with my choice. My father had to sign for me to go into the Navy since I was underage. Since they were just outside of San Francisco, the recruiter there sent a chief petty officer out to my father's house with all the paperwork. My dad told me the chief petty officer said I was probably one of the few students that didn't need a scholarship program but was very eligible for it. I didn't need it in the sense that I didn't need the money to go to school but I was most eligible for it because my grade point was 3.9.

I got promoted to ensign in November 1972. That was a highlight because Admiral Duerk, who had just become an Admiral, came out to San Francisco for the promotion. People from the Midwest also came out to San Francisco and we were promoted to ensign together.

My first duty station was Philadelphia at the height of the Vietnam conflict. I was assigned to orthopedics. In Philadelphia there were four floors of orthopedics and I was assigned between all four floors. The amputee unit was on the first floor, the hand and ENT unit on the second floor, and the third and fourth floors had the general orthopedic units. That was my first experience with nursing and what an experience it was.

It was a learning experience working with the corps staff. It's hard to believe those kids were 18, 19, 20 years old. It was interesting being on night shift and having all four floors with just one nurse and 160 patients. It was very scary now that I look back on it. I remember carrying a thousand keys in my pockets. We had antiquated narcotic lockers with a red light in them that we had to get on a stool to reach.

I remember the four floors of orthopedic patients and trying to get all the pre-op patients ready for surgery by six o'clock in the morning. They had to be up, showered and all the charts and lab work together. One time I was the only one on nights. There were so many patients going to the OR, I thought that the best thing for me to do was to get all the first cases ready to go. I think there were seven of them. I got those seven ready and left the rest for the day shift. I will never forget being "chewed out" by the charge nurse for not having all 17 prepped and ready to go. I said, "But I couldn't get it all done. There was just so much to do." I was in the stairwell with my arms wrapped around the banister because I was ready to punch her. One of the physicians came up, realized what was going on and got another department head to come and basically split us up. I was told to just go home and she would deal with it.

I was in Philly from 1973 to 1975. In 1975, I was shipped to Guam. I was put on a 30-day notice to be shipped out to help with the evacuation of South Vietnam. The evacuees were coming to Guam for processing. I got put on three-day notice. I was given all these shots and I was sicker than a dog. They had to give them to us all together since they didn't know when we were going to leave. I had typhoid, typhus, cholera, plague, yellow fever, and a couple of others, nine all together. I was sick for about five days.

After 30 days they took us off the roster to go. I was off the list for a week and then got a phone call saying I was going to leave the next day, be packed and ready to go. I closed up my apartment and gave my cat to one of the other nurses who had a family to take care of it. I had given a friend of mine the power of attorney to pay my bills and keep the apartment going. I was literally shipped off in 24 hours.

I and three corpsmen left Philly and flew to Chicago, where we picked up 50 other people. While in Chicago, I called my parents and told them I was going to have a six-hour layover in San Francisco. I didn't know when I would be back, and asked if they wanted to come see me at the airport. They did come. There were about 75 to 100 of us when we got there from all over the country. We all boarded a United Airline flight and went to Hawaii, where we picked up more people. There were a lot of us working on the units from all over the country. By the time we got to Guam, we had about 175 of us.

We landed at Anderson Air Force Base on Guam and got bused down to the hospital. We landed about 3:30 in the morning and got to the hospital about 3:45. The chief nurse basically told us we were going to be working three shifts. There were a lot of us working on the units from all over the country. The day shift and evening shift were going to work ten hours and the night shift was going to work eight. We were given quarters and literally the room was a bunk bed. There were no curtains on the windows, it was hot, and it was dirty. We had a van and went to the commissary to pick up cleaning supplies. We spent most of the day cleaning and putting sheets and tin foil up on the windows. I had to work that night from 10

P.M. to 8 A.M., so I slept for a couple of hours before heading off for my first shift.

We had an open-bay ward. There were two sections of the ward. One was an open-air solarium that had bunk beds and the other was an open ward with the old metal crank beds so we put blankets on the floor underneath the beds because we had so many patients.

The first night we admitted 30 people. I had never started an IV or put in a foley catheter or put down an NG tube. I was the med and treatment nurse that night. I put in 30 IVs and I put in 15 or 20 Foley catheters because these patients were dehydrated. Some of them came in with some very exotic diseases. Some had malaria, typhoid, typhus, and one or two might have had cholera. We had a 12-year-old girl on the ward that had tapeworms. They were so bad they had gotten in her lungs. I will never forget because they said if she started coughing you need to grab some gloves and run because she would be coughing up a tapeworm and it would choke her. We literally would have to go and help her by pulling out a worm.

Over the course of three months we had 598 patients come through our unit alone. We literally saw everything. We had one patient who had been on board a military transport ship. It was a young boy who had developed seizures and had a cardiac arrest. They brought him to us and we put him on a ventilator. He eventually did pass away. His father had been very rich and he tried to offer us money to keep his son alive. They were very religious, too. The father cut off his own hair in an offering to the gods to help save his son. I have a letter that the father wrote, thanking us for the care we provided to his son.

We were on a hill overlooking Agana, the capital of Guam. In order for planes to land in Agana they flew over the hospital. This caused the patients to scatter because they were scared to death it was a bomb. They would just huddle in corners. On the pediatric unit the Corps of Engineers built boxes on stilts that could be used as cribs. The families would not let the nurses keep their babies in these cribs because they looked like coffins. I have pictures of babies on the floor in blankets. The only time these babies were in these boxes was when the nurses had to provide care for them.

If Vietnam refugee mothers were pregnant and within three months of delivery, they were kept on Guam until they delivered because we didn't want to fly them. The mothers and their families were kept together at a little camp called Asan. When the mother was ready to deliver, she would come to the hospital. We had one mother who had five boys and delivered another boy and another mother who had five girls and had delivered another girl. When we went to discharge one of the patients, we matched armbands, and "low and behold," the patient had the wrong baby. We couldn't figure it out and so we took the baby back to the nursery and got the right baby. We went to discharge the patient and once again she had the wrong baby. We got an interpreter and found out that the mother that had all girls didn't need another girl; she needed a son to take care of the family. The one with all boys didn't need another boy, and so they just swapped babies. This was a normal cultural thing to them. Since the babies were born on United States property and essentially in the United States, we couldn't just swap babies. We kept both families for a couple days and had a complete legal adoption.

Once the babies were delivered, we shipped the families to one of the three holding points in the United States, one of which was Camp Pendleton. There were several camps across the United States. Eventually the families were dispersed through churches and family organizations throughout the community. There was one person I met who was a refugee and became a nurse. I actually was working with her at Kaiser Permanente Medical Center in San Francisco.

When the experience on Guam was concluded, I came back to Philadelphia. Because of all the experience I had had, they put me in the surgical ICU and I was there for a year and a half. I did not like the experience at all. It was just too fast paced and scary for me. The patients were just really sick and I didn't have the stamina for that kind of care. A year and a half later I got transferred to a different unit.

One of the things I remember about my ICU time was when we had a death. The patient was on active duty status. He was brought into the SICU on a ventilator. We knew he was not going to make it and it was decided to retire him. In order for his family to receive benefits he had to be retired and live until the process was complete. We needed to keep him alive until after midnight when his retirement would kick in. I remember that by 10 we knew it was going to be really touch and go. We did everything we possibly could. We put him on an external pacemaker, kept him on the vent, kept the IVs going. His retirement kicked in at midnight and we kept him going until about two in the morning just to make sure that everything was okay. When it appeared there would be no question about

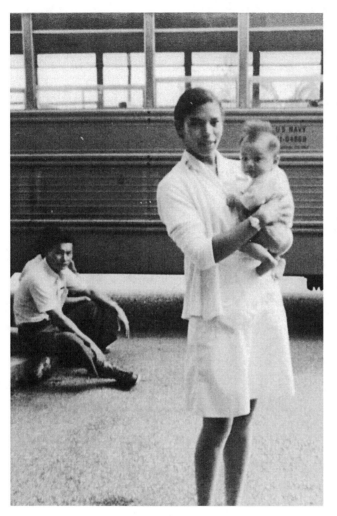

Odette P. Willis in Guam.

the retirement, we turned everything off and he died immediately. It was just the idea that what we were doing was to help the family. That will stick in my mind forever. I've actually seen and heard of it being done quite often just to ensure the family will get the retirement. This guy was in for over 20 years and was eligible for full retirement.

We had a patient come in after a motorcycle accident. He'd hit something and flew off of the motorcycle but didn't let go of the handle bars. He landed back on the motorcycle right over the gas can. When he was brought in his scrotum was swollen to the size of a basketball. It was very difficult to find a penis to put a folly catheter in. He survived.

The third thing that happened while I worked in the SICU, a friend of my family's came in for surgery. Because he had a cardiac history, they were worried he wasn't going to do very well. We brought him into cardiac ICU and did pre-op teaching along with his family. I happened to be on that day and taught the family. He had his surgery and I was able to take care of him. That was something they will never forget because I talked to the family and they said, "We'll never forget how well you took care of us."

I was sent from surgical ICU to psych and really enjoyed it. I was there for nine months and I was the charge nurse for the rehab psych unit. Margaret Whitecell was the department head. She was rough and gruff but a real "teddy bear." I learned a lot of my management skills from her as she mentored me. The biggest thing I remember about my psych experience was when we had a young marine, 19, 20 years old, come in who had been stationed on a ship. We didn't know what caused it but this guy went schizophrenic. He was so ill I will never forget him. We were giving him two to three hundred milligrams of thorazine an

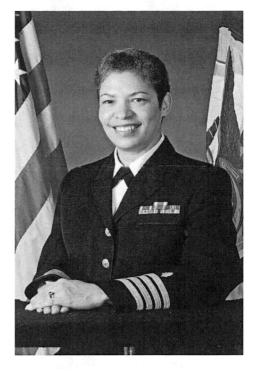

Odette P. Willis at retirement.

hour. We gave him 5 ml of Haldol every two to three hours. Nothing would touch this guy. We kept him in isolation. He would walk and walk and bang his head against the wall, or he would rock and rock. It took five days of round the clock medication to finally get him to fall asleep. He didn't sleep for five solid days. Finally, when we got him to lie down long enough to sleep, we were able to start working with him. Eventually he was transferred to a VA hospital. When we did transfer him, he was beginning to come around. I've never seen such high doses given with no effect at all. You give someone a hundred mg of Thorazine; they'll sleep for a week. This guy was getting a hundred to two hundred an hour. It was insane.

My biggest thing about Philadelphia was when I was Nurse of the Day (NOD) for the whole hospital. I was just a lieutenant! I will never forget because it was my birthday, December 1. It was a common statement made by folks who had nothing to lose to say, "Well, they can't take away my birthday." On this December 1, I kept saying, "People are wrong, they can take away your birthday." I was the NOD and it started snowing on the evening shift. The military nurses had to come in but the civilian nurses were calling in sick. I had to rearrange the staffing in order to prevent a shortage. It worked out because I kept a couple of OB nurses over to work a double shift. I told them they could sleep as long as there were no patients coming in. If one more nurse had called in sick, I would have had to work that whole shift too.

I was transferred to Cherry Point, North Carolina, in 1977 and was the charge nurse for family medicine, basically females and pediatrics. It was a good experience. I was the only military nurse on night shift in the whole hospital. We had corpsmen and the civilian nurses that were on OB and in the nursery. It was full service but we had only 90 beds. If there was a "double header" in the OB, you would have to go and help with the second delivery. If there were more babies in the nursery than they could handle, you would have to go and help with that. On the weekends you were literally the OR nurse. If a patient came in and needed that OR, you did all the prep work, the circulating, and then you recovered the patient. Because I had the ICU experience, if we had an ICU patient, then I would end up providing the care.

I attended pediatrics resuscitation codes. One was a four-day-old baby and one was a twelve-month-old. CPR really works because both of the babies pinked up as we provided it. They wouldn't breath on their own and the minute you stopped, they stopped. We lost both of them. The four-day-old was a T4 deficiency and the mother had lost a baby earlier to the same thing. At that time they weren't doing genetic testing or counseling. They were assuming that probably all of her babies would end up with this deficiency so she wasn't going to be able to get pregnant again. The second baby was a 12-month-old that came in as an abused child. The father said that the baby had hung herself off of the crib railing. The railing was an inch wide and there was no way she could have got it caught behind her jaw. That baby didn't survive either. The father was arrested.

At Cherry Point I lived in the community. I bought a home because there weren't any apartments there, and they all had waiting lists. I tried to "augment" a couple of times while I was at Cherry Point so I could go back to school. I was turned down for all of it, so I had a decision to make. Do I re-enlist for another two or three years or do I just get out? I spent two weeks crying while trying to make that decision. One day I woke up and I said, "I know exactly what I need to do. I love teaching corpsmen and I wanted to teach." So I decided to get off active duty and I applied and was accepted to UCLA in the master's degree program. I went to UCLA and received my master's in nursing as a clinical specialist in acute care, adult medical-surgical nursing with a focus in nursing education. I contacted a reserve unit to try and get in but there were no billets. I then thought nothing of it. I didn't realize I was still part of the Navy. I was just IRR.

Odette graduated from UCLA with a master's degree in 1981. She stayed in the Navy reserve and eventually became a lieutenant commander. During Operation Desert Storm she was recalled to Oakland Naval Hospital for ten months. After she returned from her mobilization she continued with the reserve and was involved in a number of military field exercises, helping to put together 196 care-plan algorithms that were computerized and placed on the corpsmen's PDAs so that the corpsmen could use them to care for patients in the field. Odette was stationed at the Bureau of Medicine and Surgery in Washington, D.C., as the reserve corps liaison. She acted as the commanding officer of several naval reserve units and retired from the Navy as a captain. As a civilian she has worked as a systems analyst and nurse educator, and now holds a full-time faculty position in the School of Nursing at George Mason University.

References

Doyle, E., and S. Lipsman. 1982. *Setting the Stage: The Vietnam Experience*. 25 vols. Boston: Boston Publishing Company.

Hovis, B. 1992. *Station Hospital Saigon: A Navy Nurse in Vietnam, 1963–1964*. Annapolis, MD: Naval Institute Press.

Nurses in the Vietnam War. 1995. *Nebraska Nurse: The Official Publication of the Nebraska Nurses Association* 28 (2, no. 2) (1995): 1, 4.

Roark, J. L., M. P. Johnson, P. C. Cohen, S. Stage, A. Lawson, and S. M. Hartmann. 1998. *The American Promise: A History of the United States from 1865*. Vol. 2. Boston: Bedford Press.

Ruff, Cheryl L., and K. Sue Roper. 2005. *Ruff's War*. Annapolis, MD: U.S. Naval Institute Press.

Rushton, P. 2010. *Gulf War Nurses: Personal Accounts of 14 Americans, 1990–1991 and 2003–2010*. Jefferson, NC: McFarland.

Rushton, P., L. C. Callister, and M. Wilson. 2005. 1998. *Latter-day Saint Nurses at War: A Story of Caring and Sacrifice*. Provo: Religious Studies Center, Brigham Young University.

www.vietnam-war.info/facts/facts3.php. Accessed August 27, 2011.

Index

Index

Index

Ricks College 90
Rolling Thunder 106
Rutgers University 76

St. Joseph's Hospital School of Nursing
  151
St. Mary's Hospital, San Francisco 65
St. Therese School of Nursing 157
St. Vincent's Hospital 151
USS *Sanctuary* 44, 48, 49, 50, 60, 81,
  145, 164
Schering-Plough Pharmaceuticals 74
Seattle University 154
Shellback 155
Sisters of Mercy 64
USS *Solace* 81
Stack, Robert 74
State University of New York 17
Surgical Hospital, 18th 60, 62, 139
Swedish Hospital School of Nursing 55

Tet Offensive 114, 132, 145, 152
Texas Woman's University 171
Titulinka 83
Todd, C. Edwina 143, 150
Truman, Harry S. 1

United States Agency for International
  Development 12

University of Arizona 160
University of California at Los Angeles
  181
University of Maryland School of Nurs-
  ing 99, 131
University of Michigan 107, 111
University of North Carolina at Chapel
  Hill School of Public Health 96
University of San Francisco 64, 68
University of Utah 167

Veterans Hospital, Minneapolis 135
Victory in Europe Day 82
Vietnam Veterans Association 63
Vietnam Women's Memorial 5, 21, 105,
  141
Vita Blue 163

Walter Reed Army Institute of Nursing
  (WRAIN) 94, 95, 96, 99
Wangensteen suction 83
Wathen, Jane 110
Westmoreland, William Childs 87
White House 18
Whitecell, Margaret 179
William Beaumont General Hospital
  56

187